PATIENT

SATISFACTION

Understanding and Managing

the Experience of Care

Second Edition

PATIENT
SATISFACTION

Understanding and Managing

the Experience of Care

Second Edition

Irwin Press

Health Administration Press
ACHE Management Series

10   09   08   07   5   4   3   2

Library of Congress Cataloging-in-Publication Data

Press, Irwin.
    Patient satisfaction : understanding and managing the experience of care / Irwin Press.—2nd ed.
        p. cm.
    Previous ed. has subtitle: Defining, measuring, and improving the experience of care.
    Includes bibliographical references.
    ISBN-13: 978-1-56793-250-8 (alk. paper)
    ISBN-10: 1-56793-250-9 (alk. paper)
    1. Patient satisfaction.   2. Physician and patient.   3. Medical care—Quality control.   I. Title.
    R727.3.P725 2005
    362.1068—dc22   2005054579

The paper used in this publication meets the minimum requirements of American National Standard for Information Sciences—Permanence of Paper for Printed Library Materials, ANSI Z39.48-1984. ⊚™

Acquisitions manager: Audrey Kaufman; Project manager: Amanda Karvelaitis; Cover designer: Betsy Pérez

Health Administration Press
A division of the Foundation of the
    American College of Healthcare Executives
1 North Franklin Street, Suite 1700
Chicago, IL 60606-3424
(312) 424-2800

Contents

Foreword: The Emerging Context of Patient Satisfaction

Ian Morrison, Ph.D.

EVERYONE WILL TELL you that the patient is at the center of healthcare. Doctors, nurses, and hospital CEOs tell you, "We put the patient first." Even strategy consultants put the patient at the center of their PowerPoint™ slides. But to put the patient first requires discipline by both caregivers and institutions. Simply saying it does not make it so.

Over the last 30 years, a new science has emerged: measuring and then managing the patient's experience of care. This new science provides the discipline needed to *really* put the patient first.

Irwin Press, Ph.D., has been a pioneer in this new field as thinker, teacher, leader, and entrepreneur. Press and his colleagues have built the intellectual and service infrastructure used to measure and manage patient satisfaction in healthcare. His deep research base and practical insights are invaluable to those who want to improve the patient's experience. This book is particularly timely because of four key trends in the healthcare marketplace: new consumers, consumer-deflected healthcare, the rise of transparency in cost and quality, and transformational purchasing.

NEW CONSUMERS

While much nonsense has been written and spoken regarding the consumer in healthcare, it is undeniable that there are powerful forces making the consumer more central as both demanding patient and reluctant payer. Baby-boom patients and those caring for or advising aging parents are more skeptical and demanding than previous generations; they want and expect high levels of service from institutions. The generations that follow are even more demanding; they are online, plugged-in, and difficult to please. Healthcare institutions need to take the pulse of these emerging consumers and respond intelligently to their needs, wants, and aspirations.

CONSUMER-DEFLECTED HEALTHCARE

The trend toward patient as payer of healthcare, couched in the language of consumer-directed healthcare, is perhaps the most important. The idea is to deflect the responsibility for payment and decision making in healthcare toward the consumer. Consumer copayments, deductibles, and premium sharing are on the rise. New plan designs, such as health savings accounts and so-called consumer-directed health plans, are leading indicators for a broader trend toward high-deductible health plans. Primary care is turning retail, and while hospital care is covered for catastrophic cases, there are a lot of deductibles and cost-sharing gimmicks on the way to full coverage.

All of these cost-shifting arrangements are forcing consumers to make choices. The best plans and benefit designs provide some tools to judge the price and quality trade-offs, but they are still inadequate. The worst designs force significant noncompliance for those with chronic illness and create an irritating and sometimes financially devastating "gotcha" when poor patients finally find out how much they really owe. One thing I know from 20 years of survey research with my partners at Harris Interactive and Harvard University is that when consumers pay more out of pocket, they get very cranky with the healthcare system in general; this spills over into their satisfaction with care. Improving patients' experience of how we bill and collect, communicate prices and share costs, and manage their expectations when real consumer dollars change hands will become ever more critical in the future.

THE RISE OF TRANSPARENCY IN COST AND QUALITY

The confluence of three powerful forces is fueling the rise of transparency in cost and quality. First are the aforementioned trends toward consumer responsibility for payment and decision making. You cannot ask consumers to choose without providing them with information on which to base the choices. (By the way, the tools today are woefully inadequate, particularly in measuring the cost part of the calculus.)

Second is the rise of the quality movement. From Six Sigma to the National Quality Forum, from the Institute for Healthcare Improvement to the National Committee on Quality Assurance, pioneering initiatives have helped us turn the corner on the measurement and reporting of cost and quality of health plans, hospitals, nursing homes, and individual providers. Providers fought this kicking and screaming—or passively aggressively at best—but the momentum is such that we will not go back to a healthcare system where decisions are made solely on blind trust or a hunch, unencumbered by evidence.

Third, and perhaps most important, is the big dog, CMS, the artist formerly known as HCFA, which has embraced measurement and reporting and will embed such measures in future payment streams (more below). All of these trends toward transparency of quality and cost measures make the measurement and management of patient satisfaction more important than ever before. The need is even more acute because, as this book clearly shows, patient satisfaction, clinical performance, institutional excellence, and overall quality are all closely correlated.

TRANFORMATIONAL PURCHASING

Large purchasers, both public and private, are using their purchasing clout and their ability to engage individual patients through benefit designs (as levers and agents) to transform healthcare delivery. This is taking the form of pay-for-performance initiatives, where provider reimbursement is tied to specific performance measures of clinical care and patient satisfaction. This is also seen in the emerging tiered-network products, where consumers will be given financial incentives to select providers and hospitals based on their measured clinical quality and efficiency. Patients will be given a financial break if they use the more efficient providers (sounds like managed care in the 1980s, eh?). But this time, so the argument goes, health plans are selecting the "most efficient" based not only on the depth of the price discounts but also on the quality and satisfaction measures, as well as on the longitudinal analysis of the provider's overall use and cost of healthcare for a given set of conditions. The broader intent of all these transformational purchasing initiatives is to encourage the healthcare delivery system to improve in terms of cost, quality, and patient satisfaction. Therefore, we will need clear and defensible scorecards for the new world that measure and report all the elements of the emerging calculus from price to patient satisfaction.

This book is both timeless and timely. It is timeless in that Irwin Press knows the patient satisfaction business better than anyone else. But it is also particularly timely because of the trends described above. If the patient is truly going to be at the center of healthcare, we need to measure and manage their experience, not just pass the burden to them and hope they don't notice.

Preface to the Second Edition

THIS SECOND EDITION offers some significant new material. A new chapter on cultural competence deals with the ways in which hospitals can manage both diverse patients and staff. Another new chapter offers 50 easy ideas for improving patients' hospital experience. There are new chapter segments on patient safety, physician satisfaction, complaint management, and scripting. The basic message, however, will never change: A concern for patient satisfaction is good for all constituencies.

A few words on how to use the book: The first two chapters are devoted to justifying why serious attention must be paid to patient satisfaction. These chapters should be mandatory reading by all. Staff will be far more committed to your satisfaction programs when they can fully appreciate that both their mission and their jobs are significantly dependent on patient perceptions and evaluations of care. Chapters 3 and 4 dig beneath the surface for insight to the roots of patient satisfaction. Nurses, physicians, technologists, and other front line staff will benefit from understanding that satisfaction is the product of interaction between two cultures—patient and hospital. What patients want from care is far more than smiles and introductions. It is a complex business. Chapter 10, contributed by consultant Mary Malone, offers 50 proven examples of satisfaction-enhancing ideas from hospitals across the country. Chapter 11 offers insight into the complex nature of the emergency department visit. The rest of the chapters will be of particular relevance to those who direct and implement your patient satisfaction programs. These chapters reflect two basic concepts: (1) You cannot manage well what you do not measure well; and (2) Measurement alone is not management. We look at how to analyze your patient survey data to get maximum insight into the sources of satisfaction and dissatisfaction. We then look at ideas and techniques for improving the patient's experience of care.

Since the first edition of the book appeared several years ago, national discussions of patient satisfaction have heated up. The Joint Commission on Accreditation of Healthcare Organizations (JCAHO) requires hospitals to monitor satisfaction. The Centers for Medicare & Medicaid Services (CMS) has finally developed its Hospital Consumer Assessment of Health Plans Survey (HCAHPS) with the expectation that hospitals will use it for public reporting of patient satisfaction levels.

"Pay for performance" is an evolving concept. External entities may look at hospital quality in calculating reimbursements. Internally, growing numbers of hospitals are using patient satisfaction scores in decisions regarding staff compensation and bonuses. Some hospitals are holding outside venders, such as food service or housekeeping contractors, responsible for maintaining high satisfaction scores and are tying a portion of the contract price to survey results. Nationally and publicly, concern for satisfaction is socially and politically correct.

Of all the reasons for paying attention to patient satisfaction, only one transcends correctness, accountability, or accreditation standards—quality of care. Patient satisfaction is important because it is a component of care as well as an outcome of care. When patients are satisfied, both the immediate care and subsequent clinical outcomes are enhanced. At the same time, when the quality of care is high, satisfaction will be measurably high. This "double whammy" should be sufficient to make improving and monitoring patient satisfaction a core concern of every healthcare institution and provider.

This is not yet the case, but it is getting better. Many still take patient satisfaction for granted as a simplistic concept that only requires common sense to understand and track. When those who believe this make little progress in improving satisfaction, their lack of success is often attributed to the soft, idiosyncratic, and unpredictable nature of patient satisfaction. Other healthcare professionals who do take patient satisfaction seriously may become frustrated by the lack of clear improvement and frequently blame the survey.

This book is directed to all who wish to improve the patient's experience and evaluation of care and who are willing to put some sweat equity into the effort. Patient satisfaction is not simple. If it were, then all hospitals would have high scores. If merely smiling, introducing yourself, and personally taking patients and guests to their destinations were all that mattered, then satisfaction would be universally high. But the patient's experience and evaluation of care involve far more than these obvious surface tactics.

That is what this book is about—the often-missed factors that underlie patient satisfaction and its management.

The patient is with you for a relatively short time—hours or days. There is no time to educate the patient to understand or appreciate what you are doing; therefore, total responsibility for satisfying the patient lies with you. The key to patient satisfaction lies in: (1) understanding the patient, (2) understanding yourself and your hospital's culture, and (3) effectively utilizing your survey data.

Most chapters end with a list of specific suggestions entitled "Action for Satisfaction." Many chapters include examples of survey results and analyses that show the usefulness of good satisfaction data. Most hospitals have access to similar data, whether internally or externally generated. These data were drawn from Press Ganey Associates surveys and reports, but most patient satisfaction survey firms provide similar analyses; if you do your own programming and data crunching, you can generate similar reports.

Healthcare has changed a lot since 1983, when I first started lecturing on patient satisfaction. The three biggest changes from my perspective are the (1) rise of the concern for quality, (2) empowerment of the patient as consumer, and (3) providers' concern for the bottom line and market share. Patient satisfaction has a major effect on all three. I hope this volume adequately supports your need to deal effectively with these issues.

While a number of specific case studies from specific hospitals about techniques or strategies can be used to improve patient satisfaction, I have tried not to overdo my representation of case studies. The problem with a specific case study is that the issue and action depicted may not be relevant for all readers. Thus, I present these as examples only, to stimulate creative discussion rather than to offer a definitive solution.

This is a very personal book and my biases are likely very apparent. I am an unflinching advocate for patient satisfaction and a firm believer that it is inextricably linked with the true quality of care. The distinction between technical and interpersonal care, or between care and service, should be laid to rest once and for all. Every one of the patient's experiences in the hospital (i.e., those with people, machines, or events) are filtered through the patient's knowledge, personality, prejudices, preconceptions, and culture. These filters determine the patient's ultimate evaluation of the experiences, and this evaluation in turn affects the patient's response to care. Mind and body are not wholly independent entities. What the patient experiences, feels, believes, thinks, fears, and hopes about care cannot be separated from the actual outcome of care. Thus, concern for patient satisfaction must ultimately become a routine part of medical management—a day-to-day concern no less important than infection control and surgical protocols. I suspect that this passion of mine will be very apparent throughout the book!

Acknowledgments

SPECIAL THANKS TO Mel Hall, Dennis Heck, Carla Peterson, and Bob Wolosin for their critical readings of earlier drafts. Thanks to Mary Malone for contributing a chapter to this second edition. Thanks to my partner, Rod Ganey, for his wisdom and suggestions. Thanks to Charlene Murphy and Deb Notestine for their help in editing my drafts. Thanks to my wife, Andra, for her support and inspiration. Amanda Karvelaitis and Audrey Kaufman of the Health Administration Press deserve thanks for making the editing process so author friendly. Above all, I am grateful to the Press Ganey family of hospital clients who continually rejuvenate me with their passion for improving the quality of care.

CHAPTER 1

Justifying the Effort: Patient Satisfaction and the Quality of Care

SATISFYING PATIENTS TAKES serious effort. So, why bother with it? There are loads of reasons. In sum, patient satisfaction can be a core strategy for achieving and sustaining the mission of your institution. When you take patient satisfaction very seriously,

- you will achieve higher quality of care;
- your staff will be more content with their jobs, and turnover will be lower;
- you will be more likely to stay financially healthy;
- your competitive position will be strengthened; and
- you will be less likely to be sued.

Patient satisfaction is a hot topic. Everyone pays lip service to it. It's politically correct. The Joint Commission says you have to monitor patient satisfaction, and it can also satisfy ORYX requirements. The National Committee for Quality Assurance (NCQA) requires HMOs to monitor it. The Centers for Medicare & Medicaid Services (CMS) has developed the Hospital Consumer Assessment of Health Plans Survey (HCAHPS) that it wants hospitals to use as a public patient satisfaction report card. State hospital associations are including patient satisfaction in their public report cards. Increasingly, purchasing coalitions and businesses will require providers to monitor it. So, you have to do something about patient satisfaction. But what?

THE CARE VERSUS SERVICE FALLACY

In spite of the books, articles, and hype, possibly no element in healthcare is so little understood as patient satisfaction. Many still view it as a soft phenomenon—a happy camper index that reflects medically uneducated perceptions as opposed to serious evaluations of real quality. Many healthcare professionals still feel that patients may be able to judge service but not technical/medical care. If the food is bad, then they might rate the whole spectrum of care lower. Service and care are distinct entities, they might contend. Do not confuse the two. *Care*—direct technical intervention (emphasis on "technical")—is the key. *Service* is peripheral—interpersonal and experiential. To such professionals, "service" suggests that you are treating customers rather than patients. This insults their professional identity.

Service is often viewed as a matter of personality and amenities. Such views have led to simplistic approaches to dealing with patient satisfaction. Most service-focused programs have not changed much from the guest-relations efforts of the 1980s, which staff often labeled as "smile school." Look the patient in the eye when talking. Introduce yourself. Sit next to the patient rather than stand at the foot of the bed. Be courteous. Be caring (whatever that means). Be prompt. Reduce delays. Keep the soup hot and the carpets clean. Care, on the other hand, is often viewed as having to do with IV hook-ups, medication, treatment explanations, postoperative instructions, and other technical or informational interventions.

In truth, the service/care distinction is a red-herring issue. It's all service, and it's all care. The manner in which care is delivered defines, for the patient, the nature and effectiveness of that care.

Timeliness, attitudes, information, explanations, body language, physical touch, contextual sounds and sights—all these factors have an effect on the patient's experience of care.

If patients perceive the carpets to be soiled, or corridor noise excessive, or the nurses less than friendly, then will it affect their experience of care? Notice I said "experience" of care, not care itself. The difference is significant. From the patient's perspective, care involves *everything* that goes on, everything that is experienced. Every vista, sound, interaction, and intervention contributes to the overall experience and is interpreted as a purposeful aspect of care. No patient wants to think that *anything* unplanned happens in a hospital.

The patient is in a strange place with strange and anxiety-producing rituals. Stress is common. Disorientation is common. If the nurse fails to provide adequate reassurance or information as she attempts to insert the IV, is this an issue of service or care? If her appearance, body language, or manner do not communicate empathy as she sticks the patient, is this a care or service issue? What about food? For many patients, the simple, familiar, nurturing ritual of meal time provides some feeling of groundedness. If the meal is delayed or if it is unattractively prepared, is this a failure of service or care? Again, to the patient, there is no way to distinguish between the two. Everything the hospital or clinic does is defined as care.

What do patients want from healthcare—technical quality or service quality? Unless asked directly, they usually will not contribute information about what they want (Baker 1998, 72). In a study by the Voluntary Hospitals of America (VHA 2000, 19), patients were asked whether clinical quality or service quality carried more weight in their healthcare decision making. Of the respondents, 32 percent said service was more important, while 68 percent ranked clinical quality more highly. When the choices were expanded to include clinical quality, service quality, or both, fully 59 percent of the initial 68 percent said they would prefer both, while 32 percent steadfastly continued to stress service over clinical quality. All things being equal, we all want the highest quality of technical (clinical) care. Technical care is a necessary criterion for judging care overall. At the same time, it is only a partial—and thus insufficient—criterion for making this judgment.

Patients do judge the quality of clinical care they receive. However, they base their judgments on far more than the technical interventions, many of which they are unaware. Patients cannot judge whether the proper gauge needle is being used for the injection, whether 10 cc is the proper dose, or whether heparin is the proper medication. But patients can judge whether the injection hurt more than anticipated, whether the nurse was informative as well as friendly, or whether the doctor listened to the patient's ideas and questions and responded appropriately.

Patients cannot distinguish between the technical merits of full incision versus endoscopic surgery for hernia repair, but they can judge whether the doctor explained the options well. They can judge whether staff were sensitive to their postoperative pain or whether friends and visiting family were treated with respect and given satisfactory explanations. Patients are aware of whether sensitive, realistic information was given about care at home after discharge or whether the staff appeared to empathize with the personal hardships that resulted from the physical problem and the hospitalization.

Patients enter an interaction with physicians assuming—or at least hoping—that they are competent. However, if patients perceive that physicians are not interested in them or are not concerned with good communication or empathy, then they doubt the physicians' ability to actually use their full competence (Freidson 1961, 208–9). Patients would then feel that the care being delivered was not of the highest quality. Moreover, they would likely respond with some level of distrust, potentially resulting in an incomplete information exchange and a less-than-optimal response to treatment.

In short, the patient's perception of the physician's technical competence could actually modify the effectiveness of that competence. Here again, service and care are inseparable. The patient's total experience of care defines that care and affects the patient's response to it. That this experience is highly personal actually makes its effect on the patient even stronger (e.g., Goldfield et al. 1999, 430). The interactional and perceptual aspect of the experience and the inclusion of familiar service elements, as well as technical interventions, make the experience no less significant as a definer of quality.

Patients' experiences and perceptions of care are expressed and measured as patient satisfaction. Therefore, patient satisfaction is a valid outcome indicator of the quality of the totality of care experienced.

CARE VERSUS CURE

What if a patient has a lousy, dissatisfying experience in the hospital yet has a good technical outcome? What does this say about the relationship between care and cure? If there is a disconnection between patient satisfaction and clinical outcome, then what are the implications for the hospital's mission? Why bother satisfying patients?

Many disorders are self-limiting, meaning patients will recover with or without care. Care itself often does not cure. Some patients receive care designed to yield only a diagnosis (e.g., blood work, scans, biopsy), not a direct cure. For others, care is anticipated to result only in palliation of discomfort or temporary remission of symptoms. Some care is given to minimize impairment, with no hope of a return to normal. End-of-life care certainly is designed not to cure but to minimize discomfort and maximize the temporary quality of life of the patient—with death (not cure) the inevitable outcome. Care for other patients does result in an intended and ostensibly permanent remission of disease, dysfunction, or symptoms. This is the pure manifestation of cure and the ideal but frequently unrealized goal of care.

No one—no hospital, no physician—can guarantee cure. The medical problem (e.g., infection, impairment, organ failure), the patient's age, condition, life style, habits, personality, and support systems all can affect the ultimate outcome. But the hospital *can* guarantee *care*. Care includes technical intervention, empathy, information, and concern for the patient's emotional and physical comfort. Care is totally within the hospital's control.

If patients are highly satisfied with care in the broadest sense, then the most manageable part of the hospital's mission is achieved. *If a hospital's patients are dissatisfied with care, then that care is of lower quality, regardless of subsequent technical outcome.*

THE LINK TO QUALITY

In 2004, Robert Wood Johnson University Hospital in Hamilton Township, New Jersey (RWJ-Hamilton), won the prestigious Malcolm Baldrige Award. Christy Stephenson, RWJ-Hamilton's president and CEO, states that strong attention to patient satisfaction and effective use of survey data played a significant role in their being selected.

Steiber (1988, 84) reports a solid correlation (.71) between patient satisfaction and overall quality of care. Davies and Ware (1987) find a high correlation between the patients' evaluations of the technical quality of their care and clinical experts' judgments of this same care. Nelson and his colleagues (Nelson et. al 1992) find that patients' and physicians' ratings of hospital quality are highly correlated (.52 to .87). Many researchers also believe that patients are quite capable of judging the technical quality of care (Chang et al. 1984; Gerbert and Hargreaves 1986; Cleary and McNeil 1988).

What is it that allows patients to evaluate technical care? After all, patients are not competent clinicians. The consensus is that patients constantly judge the motives and competence of caregivers through their interactions with them. As indicated earlier, this judgment is a very personal one, based on perceptions of care being responsive to patients' individual needs rather than to any universal code of standards (McGlynn 1997). When these individual needs are perceived as being met, better care results. Lohr (1997, 23) notes that "Inferior care results when health professionals lack full mastery of their clinical areas or *cannot communicate effectively and compassionately*" (emphasis added). In short, when patients perceive motives, communication, empathy, and clinical judgment positively, they will respond more positively to care. This includes physical and behavioral responses to care, not just emotional or evaluational responses. Sobel (1995) claims that improved communication and interaction between caregiver and patient improves actual outcome. Donabedian (1988, 1744) notes that " . . . the interpersonal process is the vehicle by which technical care is implemented and on which its success depends" (see also Corah, O'Shea, and Bissell 1985; O'Shea, Corah, and Thines 1986; Babakus and Mangold 1992). Interpersonal and technical aspects of care are not separate phenomena.

What this boils down to is that patient satisfaction is not only an indicator of the quality of care but a *component* of quality care as well. When patients are more satisfied, four things occur regarding trust, stress, safety, and the placebo effect.

Trust Is Enhanced

Enhanced trust results in greater compliance as well as a greater tolerance of uncomfortable or frightening procedures. The relationship between interaction skills (e.g., information giving and taking, empathy) and compliance are fully documented (e.g., Ware and Davies 1984). Physicians generally are not successful at correctly identifying their compliant and noncompliant patients. Patients do not telegraph compliance. They do not usually voice complaints or question judgments on the spot, either. If patients lack trust in the care, then medical management will be more difficult and likely less effective. There can be more complaints about discomfort or fear.

...ents will also be more likely to "act out" during procedures. Staff can become frustrated.

Some years ago, I spent a year as visiting professor at a large medical school attached to the department of psychiatry. I noticed that in a majority of instances when medical residents called for a psych consult, it involved a noncompliant patient who would not follow the doctor's orders. The result was more staff intervention and, in many instances, greater resource utilization and length of stay. Overall, when patients are more satisfied, medical management is easier.

Stress Is Reduced

The relationship between stress and medical complications has been known for years (Nuckolls, Kaplan, and Cassel 1972; Crandon 1979). On the Press Ganey inpatient survey, we ask patients to rate how well their blood was drawn (e.g., quick, little pain). We also ask about the friendliness and courtesy of the phlebotomist. Not surprisingly, the two responses are significantly correlated ($r = .448$; $p < .01$). When the nurse puts a patient at ease, there is less stress, more relaxation of muscles, and an easier stick. Greater satisfaction means lower stress and less likelihood of complications.

In a fascinating study some years ago, Sosa (1983) followed a group of women who came to a large indigent hospital to deliver their first babies. All of the women in the study came to the hospital alone, with no husband or other person to accompany them. They were examined on admission and determined to have had a normal, uncomplicated pregnancy to date. All of the women were provided with standard labor/delivery care and were attended by nurses and physicians performing their normal duties. Half of the women in this sample, however, were provided with a *doula* (a supportive laywoman) to attend them during their labor and delivery.

Sosa and his colleagues found that women attended by doulas had significantly shorter labor time and experienced far fewer complications than the women who went through labor and delivery alone. Stress reduction via empathetic interaction was clearly a factor here. With increased stress, medical outcomes may be less satisfactory and higher costs are incurred because of complications.

The Placebo Effect Is Enhanced

"Placebo" is Latin for "I please." Moerman (2000) estimates that, on average, 30 percent of any cure is a result of the placebo effect. This effect is emphatically not produced by the procedure itself (i.e., the pill or technical intervention). A sugar pill is not a placebo. The *idea* of the pill and what it can do is the placebo. Every intervention in the clinical setting has a placebo effect by influencing the patient's perception of care. Information, interaction, perceived motives and attitudes of caregivers, concern for physical comfort, decor, symbols, machinery, medications, treatments—every experience contributes to the intervention. All of these can have an effect on the patient's perception of the quality and effectiveness of care while that care is being given, not just after discharge.

Physician enthusiasm, for example, can affect a patient's response to treatment. So can a confident attitude. One study of patients presenting with vague symptoms scripted doctors to use two different interactions. Doctors told one group of patients, "I don't know what's the matter with you." Patients in the other group were given a clear but benign diagnosis, such as duodenal inflammation, and were told that they needed no further treatment. Two weeks later, 39 percent of the first group reported feeling better. Sixty-four percent of the second group, which were told a definite diagnosis and prognosis, reported feeling better (Moerman 2000).

Moerman (2000) also cites studies demonstrating that short, frank preoperative discussions by anesthetists about postoperative pain led to significantly less analgesic use and shortened hospital stays for patients undergoing abdominal surgery.

The placebo effect is not limited to interactions with physicians or nurses. Any experience the patient has with the institution can exert a placebo effect. This applies to decor and food as well as surgical explanations or the courtesy of the IV nurse. With the placebo phenomenon, the effectiveness of the active intervention (i.e., the surgery or meds) is automatically enhanced. The two factors are additive, not alternatives. Patient satisfaction is a potent placebo.

SAFETY AND SATISFACTION

Yet another advantage of high patient satisfaction is the likelihood of reduced errors. This takes several forms. First, if patients are more satisfied with *general* care, then they are likely to be more trusting, less stressed, less intimidated by staff, and more collaborative during any specific aspect of care. This means that they will be more likely to ask questions and express concerns, especially if they feel something is not right. Information breeds trust and should increase patients' responsibility for their own care.

In a Press Ganey study of 564,000 patients (Wolosin 2004), a number of informational issues were examined for their correlation with the hospital's concern for the patient's safety and security. Positive and highly statistically significant correlations (at .01 level) were found between patient perceptions of their safety and the type and quality of information given during their stay. These issues involved nurses keeping the patient informed, explanations about what would happen during tests and treatments, information given to the family, and how well the physician kept the patient informed about what was going on.

Patients' perceptions of their safety in the hospital can be positively influenced if staff make gestures or statements with obvious references to safety. When the nurse washes his hands with an antiseptic wipe in front of the patient or says, "I'm checking the ID number on your wrist band to make sure we're giving you the right medicine," he is clearly demonstrating the hospital's concern for the patient's safety (for a full discussion of the link between patient satisfaction and safety, see Wolosin et al. 2006).

A most interesting finding concerned the touchy issue of information given patients upon admission about patient rights, advance directives, and organ donation. One might think that patients would be less satisfied and more worried about their safety if informed about these morbid contingencies prior to care. The contrary is true, however. Those patients who reported receiving more information about advance directives were also *more* satisfied with their overall care (Gavran 2005).

To cap this discussion, in a study of 42,000 patients at 29 midwestern hospitals, Jaipaul and Rosenthal (2003) found that hospitals with higher levels of patient satisfaction also tended to have lower mortality rates ($r = 0.40$, $p = .03$).

In sum, when patients are more satisfied, medical management and outcome are enhanced. Patient satisfaction and actual quality of care are not distinct phenomena. When your patients are more satisfied, they really are getting better care. Thus, when you measure patient satisfaction, you really are measuring your overall quality of care. *Quality of care is defined by its effect on patients, not on its being recognized as such by professional experts.*

Patients act on what they think or believe. If they think your institution is high in quality, then they will respond as though it is—regardless of the basis of their judgment.

CONCLUSIONS

We're entering a new era in health care. "Show me the quality!" will be the mantra of the new millennium. This has economic implications, of course. The core issue is still the quality of care, but this quality will no longer be taken for granted. It will be examined, measured, and put on display and will serve as the basis for public and patient decisions affecting the well-being of the hospital. CMS has already established a list of technical clinical measures that hospitals must collate and report publicly in order to receive reimbursement updates. One way or another, patient satisfaction will become fodder for public scrutiny as well.

As the patient becomes ever more a consumer, patient satisfaction becomes increasingly relevant as the key indicator of how quality of care is actually experienced by patients. Given that cure itself cannot be guaranteed, this personal experience of care—defined and measured as satisfaction—is a reasonably pure indicator of how well the hospital expresses its core mission. Satisfied patients mean higher quality care.

ACTION FOR SATISFACTION

1. Educate staff at all levels about the connection between patient satisfaction and the quality of care. This link is not intuitive. Staff must understand that the connection is direct (e.g., satisfaction and stress, compliance, information exchange) as well as indirect (e.g., a more satisfying general experience for the patient). Portions of this chapter can serve as a learning device.
2. Patient satisfaction is measured by a survey whose scores reflect staff performance as well as patient perspectives of the care delivered. Educate staff about the link between the specific survey questions and specific aspects of care.

REFERENCES

Babakus, E., and W. G. Mangold. 1992. "Adapting the SERVQUAL Scale to Hospital Services: An Empirical Investigation." *Health Services Research* 26: 767–86.

Baker, S. K. 1998. *Managing Patient Expectations*. San Francisco: Jossey-Bass.

Chang, B. L., G. C. Uman, L. S. Linn, J. E. Ware, Jr., and R. L. Kane. 1984. "The Effect of Systematically Varying Components of Nursing Care on Satisfaction in Elderly Ambulatory Women." *Western Journal of Nursing Research* 6 (4): 367–86.

Cleary, P. D., and B. J. McNeil. 1988. "Patient Satisfaction as an Indicator of Quality Care." *Inquiry* 25 (1): 25–36.

Corah, N. L., R. M. O'Shea, and G. D. Bissell. 1985. "The Dentist-Patient Relationship: Perceptions by Patients of Dentist Behavior in Relation to Satisfaction and Anxiety." *Journal of American Dental Association* 111 (3): 443–46.

Crandon, A. J. 1979. "Maternal Anxiety and Obstetric Complications." *Journal of Psychosomatic Research* 23 (2): 109–11.

Davies, A. R., and J. E. Ware, Jr. 1987. "Involving Consumers in Quality of Care Assessment: Do They Provide Valid Information?" White paper, December. Santa Monica, CA: Rand Corporation.

Donabedian, A. 1988. "The Quality of Care: How Can It Be Assessed?" *JAMA* 260 (12): 1743–48.

Freidson, E. 1961. *Patients' Views of Medical Practice: A Study of Subscribers to a Prepaid Medical Plan in the Bronx.* New York: Russel Sage Foundation.

Gavran, G. 2005. "End-of-Life Choices a Vital Part of Patient Care." *HealthLeaders News,* June 6. [Online article; retrieved 8/15/05.] http://www.healthleaders.com/news/print.php?contentid=68341.

Gerbert, B., and W. A. Hargreaves. 1986: "Measuring Physician Behavior." *Medical Care* 24 (9): 838–47.

Goldfield, N., C. Larson, D. Siegal, J. Eisenhandler, and I. Leverton. 1999. "The Content of Report Cards: Do Primary Care Physicians and Managed Care Medical Directors Know What Health Plan Members Think Is Important?" *Journal on Quality Improvement* 25 (8): 422–31.

Jaipaul, C. K., and G. E. Rosenthal. 2003. "Do Hospitals with Lower Mortality Have Higher Patient Satisfaction?" *American Journal of Medical Quality* 18 (2): 59–65.

Lohr, K. N. 1997. "How Do We Measure Quality?" *Health Affairs* 16 (3): 22–25.

McGlynn, E. A. 1997. "Six Challenges in Measuring the Quality of Care." *Health Affairs* 16 (3): 7–21.

Moerman, D. E. 2000. "Cultural Variation in the Placebo Effect: Ulcers, Anxiety, and Blood Pressure." *Medical Anthropology Quarterly* 14 (1): 51–72.

Nelson, E. C., R. T. Rust, A. Zahorik, R. L. Rose, P. Batalden, and B. A. Siemanski. 1992. "Do Patient Perceptions of Quality Relate to Hospital Financial Performance?" *Journal of Health Care Marketing* 12 (4): 6–13.

Nuckolls, K. B, B. H. Kaplan, and J. Cassel. 1972. "Psychosocial Assets, Life Crisis and the Prognosis of Pregnancy." *American Journal of Epidemiology* 95 (5): 431–41.

O'Shea , R. M., N. L. Corah, and T. J. Thines. 1986. "Dental Patients' Advice on how to Reduce Anxiety." *General Dentistry* 34 (1): 44–47.

Sobel, D. S. 1995. "Rethinking Medicine: Improving Health Outcomes with Cost-effective Psychosocial Interventions." *Psychosomatic Medicine* 57 (3): 234–44.

Sosa, R. A. 1983. "Some Observations on Effect of a Supportive Companion During Labor and Delivery." *Journal of the Florida Medical Association* 70 (9): 761–63.

Steiber, S. R. 1988. "How Consumers Perceive Health Care Quality." *Hospitals* 62 (7): 84.

Voluntary Hospitals of American (VHA). 2000. *Consumer Demand for Clinical Quality: The Giant Awakens.* 2000 Research Series, Vol. 3. Irving, TX: VHA, Inc.

Ware, J. E, Jr., and A. R. Davies. 1984. "Behavioral Consequences of Consumer Dissatisfaction with Medical Care." *Evaluation and Program Planning* 6 (3–4): 291–97.

Wolosin, R. J. 2004. "Patients' Perceptions of Safety in U.S. Hospitals." Poster presented at the AcademyHealth Annual Research Meeting, San Diego, CA, June 7–9.

Wolosin, R., L. Vercler, and J. Matthews. 2006 (in press). "Am I Safe Here?" *Journal of Nursing Care Quality.*

CHAPTER 2

Justifying the Effort:
Patient Satisfaction and
Organizational Effectiveness

THE CONCERN FOR quality alone is sufficient justification for creating a culture that thrives on patient satisfaction, but there is far more. You cannot deliver high quality care if you are out of business. To stay healthy themselves, hospitals have to attract and keep staff and physicians as well as patients. Loyalty must be earned. In this sense, staff and physicians are as much your customers as are patients. When all three constituencies are highly satisfied with your institution, your ability to meet your economic, staffing, and mission needs are maximized.

THE LINK TO EMPLOYEE SATISFACTION

If patient satisfaction were linked only to quality of care, then that would be enough to justify its importance. That patient satisfaction is also a factor in staff satisfaction—and vise versa—is an added bonus (Schlesinger and Heskett 1991). Atkins and her associates (Atkins, Marshall, and Javalgi 1996) identify a strong relationship

Figure 2.1. Relationship Between Patient Satisfaction and Employee Satisfaction

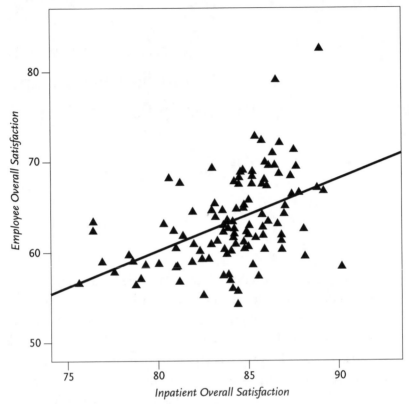

Note: r = .486; p = .01; R Sq. Linear = 0.217.
Source: Press Ganey Associates. 2005.

between employee satisfaction and patient intent to return to or recommend the hospital. In 2005, Press Ganey confirmed these findings in the largest study of its kind to date, examining the link between inpatient and employee satisfaction in 111 hospitals nationwide as shown in Figure 2.1.

These findings are hardly surprising. Any professional will be more satisfied with his or her job when sensing (or having hard data proving) that the client is pleased with his or her hard work, dedication, and service. Alternatively, patients are far more likely to have a satisfying care experience from staff who clearly get satisfaction from serving them.

A key result of staff satisfaction is reduced turnover. Thunderbird Samaritan Medical Center in Glendale, Arizona, reports that nursing staff turnover dropped from 16 percent to 11 percent from 1998 to 1999 as patient satisfaction made significant gains. Covenant Health System in Lubbock, Texas, saw employee turnover drop from 24 percent to 18 percent (a 25 percent reduction) over the two-year period in which their satisfaction scores rose significantly. Fueled by increased staff satisfaction, turnover reductions of this magnitude can mean significant savings through lower recruiting and training costs (Taylor 1999, 48). RWJ-Hamilton—a 2004 Malcolm Baldrige Award winner—reports that during the previous four years employee turnover dropped from 17 percent to 11 percent while patient satisfaction rose significantly.

Like the relationship between satisfaction and quality of care, the patient/staff satisfaction connection is natural. The linkage is not quite direct, however. Administrators and policy can act as filters—or catalysts. When staff are empowered and rewarded for behaviors and strategies that enhance patient satisfaction, both staff and patient satisfaction will likely move upward. If patient satisfaction survey scores become a club with which to threaten staff, and if staff are not rewarded for aggressively addressing identifiable satisfaction issues, then both patients and staff may find less to recommend about your institution. If patient satisfaction is high, then staff feel more pride in their work and actualize the hospital's mission more enthusiastically. High staff satisfaction is also an indicator that staff feel enabled and supported by management in fulfilling their personal missions of good patient care. The end result is more than mere job approval, of course. When provider satisfaction is high, the result is better medical treatment as well as personal care (Kurata et al. 1992).

THE LINK TO PHYSICIAN SATISFACTION

Physician loyalty to the hospital can never be taken for granted.

A 2004 Press Ganey study of 11,000 physicians at 73 hospitals nationwide examined physician satisfaction with a range of hospital characteristics (Wolosin 2004). Among the most important contributors to their satisfaction were perceived quality of the hospital and care delivered, especially how well the institutional organization and the staff facilitated the physicians' ability to deliver quality care.

Figure 2.2. Relationship Between Patient and Physician Satisfaction

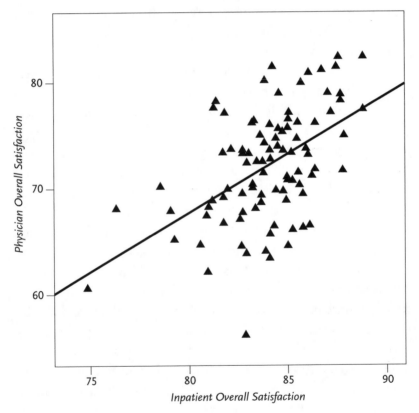

Note: r = .510; p = .01; R Sq. Linear = 0.26.
Source: Press Ganey Associates. 2005.

When physicians are more satisfied, a smooth flow of information and technical events as well as a tighter coordination of care, is reflected. Patients can sense this through the care itself and their physician's comments, tone, and attitude.

As with the relationship between patient and employee satisfaction, the high correlation between patient and physician satisfaction with the hospital is not surprising.

A 2005 Press Ganey study in 94 hospitals nationwide demonstrated a strong, statistically significant correlation between patient and physician satisfaction with the hospital, as shown in Figure 2.2.

Physicians are affected by patient satisfaction both directly and indirectly. As indicated earlier, satisfied patients are more likely to be cooperative, informative, and collaborative. This makes the physician's job easier and can have a positive impact on outcome. More indirectly, physicians are aware of the hospital's quality initiatives and patient satisfaction programs—if any. Physicians in hospitals that put significant effort into building a patient satisfaction culture and publicizing their successes are more likely to be sensitized to patients' perceptions of care.

In hospitals with higher patient satisfaction, physicians feel more positive about their own efforts, their mission, and about the whole institution.

THE LINK TO COMPETITIVE STRENGTH

Perhaps because of increasing costs, or perhaps because of the growing public familiarity with customer service in all other sectors of the economy, patients increasingly view healthcare as a commodity and are evaluating it as such. If good service is expected from McDonalds, FedEx, and Nordstrom's, then it should also be expected from the hospital that bills a thousand bucks a day. Good service should also be expected from the health plan for which employees now pay big money. Even well-insured employees are quite aware that they are paying for their own healthcare— through either reduced salaries or bigger deductions from paychecks. Healthcare is a commodity, and hospitals and health plans are advertising about as much as local car dealers do. Check out the billboards in your town.

Who is the target of the ads, billboards, fitness walks, women's health festivals, and other publicity-generating programs sponsored by most hospitals these days? The target is individual prospective patients, not physicians. Now, it could be argued that for most employed Americans of all ages, choice of hospital and physician are typically limited by the health plans they or their employers select. On the surface, this sounds like the absence of choice. But individual choice and clout are still there.

Good fringe benefits, particularly a decent health insurance plan, are becoming a potent bargaining chip for employers to use in attracting and holding desirable employees. A business owner in a mid-size southern city tells the following story.

> We have relatively low unemployment in our town. My own company won several key employees away from other local firms because of our health and sick-leave plans. We insure our employees through our health plan, a plan that offers one of four local hospitals as the in-network provider. If an employee wants to go to one of the other hospitals or other doctors, then he or she has to fork over a larger co-payment. How many valuable staff have to complain about the company plan's hospital before we decide to dump the plan for another that offers a rival institution? Certainly no more than 10 percent, and probably fewer. When we switched health plans several years ago, it was because the new plan was moderately less costly, but especially because a significant number of our staff (eight out of 100 employees) had complained about service at the previous plan's hospital. They were particularly displeased with ED staff. None of our employees complained about the switch.
>
> When we switched, the previous plan lost several hundred thousand dollars worth of business (and they did call us to find out why we took our business elsewhere). The hospital lost far more than that. At the time we switched, it lost 100 insured workers plus their average of two to three dependents. We now have over 170 insured employees.

For the hospital we no longer use, the lost opportunity cost will total in the millions of dollars over the next decade. Both cost and employee satisfaction drive our selection of health plans now. We can't afford a generalized loyalty to any particular hospital. It doesn't matter how many testimonials to their quality they publish in the local paper and on local TV or even whether their name appears among the "best hospitals in the United States" list published by a major national magazine. If enough of our employees don't like the hospital, we won't use it!

Various studies indicate how much financial loss results from a single dissatisfied patient. One patient tells 10 or 12 others, these others tell several more, and so on (see TARP 1976; Strasser and Davis 1991, 6–12). By this reckoning, those eight or ten dissatisfied employees turned off more than 120 other potential hospital customers in their town. Therefore, the hospital not only stands to lose a lot of money through a company's defection but also additional dollars through negative word of mouth that turns off a substantial number of additional potential customers (Strasser and Davis 1991, 201). The point is that individual patients are gaining unprecedented clout. Dissatisfaction can lead to significant financial consequences for the provider.

If, ultimately, patients are allowed to sue employers for service failures by the company's contracted health plan, then many firms will dodge this liability by simply giving up on selecting and offering health plans (and their providers) to employees. Companies will give employees a voucher to purchase their own insurance. These individuals will make their preferences for providers very clear to the health plans that will be competing for their business. Here, patient satisfaction becomes a key to purchase and repurchase. No organization is perfect, and hospitals are no exception. However, when customers are highly satisfied, they will be willing to reuse the facility—or another provider bearing that brand identity—even if they have had an isolated bad experience or are bombarded with public relations from a competing institution (Oliver 1996, 392).

Figure 2.3. Percentage of Americans Who Say Each Is "Very Believable" in Terms of Providing Information About Quality of Care

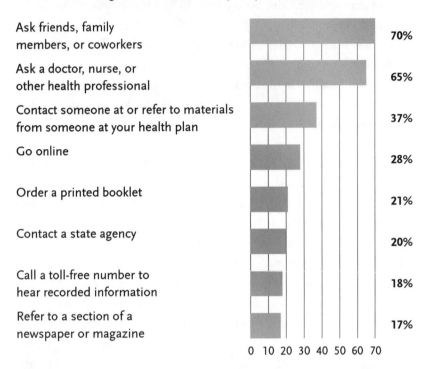

Ask friends, family members, or coworkers	70%
Ask a doctor, nurse, or other health professional	65%
Contact someone at or refer to materials from someone at your health plan	37%
Go online	28%
Order a printed booklet	21%
Contact a state agency	20%
Call a toll-free number to hear recorded information	18%
Refer to a section of a newspaper or magazine	17%

0 10 20 30 40 50 60 70

Source: Kaiser Family Foundation/Agency for Healthcare Research and Quality. 2000. *National Survey on Americans as Health Care Consumers: An Update on the Role of Quality Information.* December (conducted July 31–Oct. 13, 2000).

Truly satisfied customers become active "apostles" for the business (Jones and Sasser 1995; Gitomer 1997). Interestingly, studies find that patients are not strongly influenced by public claims of quality by hospitals or by published report cards (Tumlinson et al. 1997; Hibbard and Jewett 1997). Rather, their personal experiences and the experiences of significant others have the most effect on judgments of quality and decisions to choose one hospital over another (as shown in Figures 2.3 and 2.4). Figure 2.3 demonstrates the response when Americans were asked the question, "Who is very

Figure 2.4. Importance of Familiarity Versus Ratings

Suppose you had to choose between two hospitals

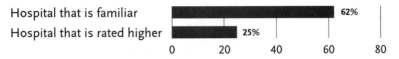

Source: Kaiser Family Foundation/Agency for Healthcare Research and Quality. 2000. *National Survey on Americans as Health Care Consumers: An Update on the Role of Quality Information.* December (conducted July 31–Oct. 13, 2000).

believable?" regarding quality of care; Figure 2.4 shows the percentage of Americans who would choose familiarity over ratings.

Ware and Davies (1984, 296) sum it up well: "In addition to delays in care seeking, in the face of serious symptoms, dissatisfaction seems to have other negative effects," including an increase in shopping around for doctors and other providers. In an era when hospitals are facing increasing competition from specialty clinics and outpatient facilities, strong patient satisfaction drives patient loyalty.

The Brand Name Phenomenon

The "hospital" is joining the dodo on the extinct list. It is being replaced by the "medical center" and the "integrated healthcare network." To compete for managed care contracts, hospitals have to offer "one-stop shopping," where a single contract will bring the payer a full line of healthcare services. Many hospitals have picked up physician practices, clinics, home health agencies, and diagnostic and surgical centers, to list a few. All of these are linked through the hospital or medical center name, which becomes the brand for the entire network. The reputations of all parts of this network are interlinked. Dissatisfaction with any one part can send patients/customers to the competitor, who probably offers a similar range of services. If Mary is dissatisfied with her experience in your emergency department (ED), then she might not want to use your outpatient surgical center next year for her hernia repair or your home health agency for her mother. Thus, the financial consequences of dissatisfied customers become multiplied.

A final word about your competition: it is not just the hospital or clinic on the other side of town. Do not forget alternative practitioners. Americans are now spending about as much on chiropractors, naturopaths, massage therapists, nutrition consultants, health food stores, and even the growing supplement sections of their corner pharmacy as they are spending on traditional healthcare. Technical excellence does not draw loyalty—and bucks—away from traditional care providers. Most people who use alternative practitioners and practices will tell you that they treat the whole person or provide a feeling of greater personal control over one's health. In truth, they provide greater patient satisfaction, not necessarily dramatic medical recoveries.

THE LINK TO PROFITABILITY

The effect of patient satisfaction goes even further. Kenagy, Berwick, and Shore (1999, 664) review a number of studies and observe "significant reductions in the costs of care when service improves." In a 51-hospital study, Nelson et al. (1992, 13) found a strong relationship between hospital financial performance and patients' ratings of care. They report that "patient-perceived quality explains up to 30 percent of the variation in hospital profitability. Relatively small increases in the level of patient satisfaction are associated with millions of dollars in year-end earnings for the average hospital" (see also Brown et al. 1993, 13, on potential loss of income to a physician practice that dissatisfies and turns away a single patient). In one of the largest studies to date, Press Ganey (2002) released findings from 679 hospitals nationwide, linking their profitability

Figure 2.5. Patient Satisfaction and Profitability

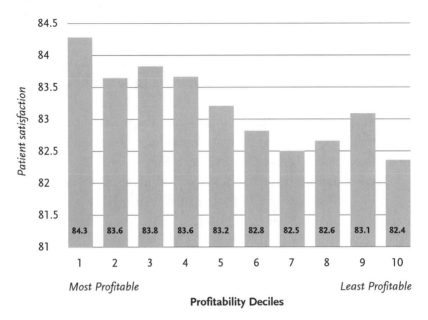

Note: r = .32; p = 0.01.
Source: Based on 2003 data from Medicare Provider Analysis and Review and Press Ganey Associates.

with patient satisfaction. A highly significant correlation was found (r = .23; p < .001) between profit and satisfaction, as shown in Figure 2.5. Data were derived from Healthcare Industries Association's (HCIA's) 2003 Medicare Provider Dataset and Press Ganey 2003 data.

Whether patient satisfaction influences financial strength or vice versa remains a question. To investigate this, Press Ganey (1998) looked at 1997 financial data from over a hundred hospitals reported by HCIA. Patient satisfaction scores from these hospitals were correlated with their profitability, and a small, statistically significant correlation was found (r = .168, significant at the .05 level). However, the really fascinating and suggestive insight emerged when we looked at these same hospitals' satisfaction scores for the years prior to 1997. We found that the 1997 profit figures were more highly correlated with patient satisfaction in 1992 (r = .269, p = .05) than in 1997! In other words, profitability is more affected by past patient satisfaction than present.

Zimmerman and Skalko (1994, 105) reach the same conclusion: Patient satisfaction is a long-term strategic tool, not just a short-term fix.

This makes good sense. Assuming that the physical problem is dealt with adequately, the patient should have no reason to return anytime soon. Three, four, or five years may elapse before the patient gives the hospital repeat business. In the meantime, he or she is paying continual verbal homage to the institution—which generates additional present-time business.

A recent study at Rush University Medical Center in Chicago, Illinois, ascertained that if patient ratings of information provided by nurses or physicians (a key satisfaction survey item) moved up from the three-to-four rating range into a four-to-five rating range on a five-item scale, then the resulting increase in return admissions would produce $2.3 million in additional patient revenue—or an additional $82 for each current patient (Garman, Garcia, and Hargreaves 2004).

The question of whether you are treating patients or customers is a red-herring issue. Many healthcare professionals cringe when they hear patients referred to as "customers." They are both. Today's patient is tomorrow's customer. The patient experiences care now, but selects and patronizes providers later as a customer. Mayer and Cates (2004, 24) offer an easy rule for deciding whether the individual you are caring for now is a patient or a customer:

> The more horizontal they are, the more they're patients.
>
> The more vertical they are, the more they're customers.

Mayer and Cates (2004, 26) estimate that 80 percent to 90 percent of patients are customers. Most patients thus start as customers. If you are doing your job well, then even those who start as patients begin their transition to being customers at some time during their stay.

Of course, a relationship does exist between present satisfaction and present profit. As we suggested earlier, satisfied patients are more likely to respond positively to treatment, have fewer complications, and so forth. This means fewer resources spent and thus a positive financial effect. If hospitals can avoid patient complaints, then resources will also be saved. Moran and Malone (1997, 64) conclude that "satisfying patients is more cost effective than responding to complaints."

Interestingly, the link between satisfaction and resource utilization is being viewed seriously by some financial institutions. Moody's Investors Service has cited improved patient satisfaction as an important factor underlying the increased revenues and market share that led to its raising a hospital's bond rating, as shown in Figure 2.6.

Figure 2.6. Moody's Investors Service Rating of Baptist Hospital

Moody's Investors Service

Baptist Hosp., Inc. & The Baptist Manor, Inc. Escambia County Health Facilities Authority, FL.

Moody's Rating	A3

Issue:
Series 1998

Sale Amount	$65,000,000
Expected Sale Date	06/24/98
Rating Description	Series 1998

Opinion:
A customer satisfaction focus, which permeates the hospital from top management down to floor personnel and whose results now serve as a benchmark for other hospitals, is making a competitive difference and reportedly contributes to some of the 9.8 percent admissions gain for the year-to-date period . . .

Source: Used with permission from Baptist Health Care Corporation, Pensacola, Florida, and Moody's Investors Service.

THE LINK TO ACCOUNTABILITY

Everyone is talking about quality, but it is more than talk. An increasing number of external entities want proof of your quality. States are making public lengths of stay and the number of C-sections physicians perform after vaginal delivery. The National Committee for Quality Assurance (NCQA) Health Plan Employer Data and Information Set (HEDIS) survey samples a hospital's quality as it taps customers' experiences with their HMOs; after all, the HMO's customers are the hospital's customers. Other agencies, payers, business coalitions, and hospital associations will be issuing report cards to the public on your performance (Kenkel 1995). CMS's HCAHPS survey is in its final stages of development. The National Quality Forum is actively attempting to identify an extensive series of outcome measures that could be implemented in all hospitals, with results reported to various public entities. Several of these report cards will likely include some form of patient satisfaction measure.

If you look bad on a report card, then your accreditation or your bottom line could be affected. An HMO, business coalition, or purchasing group may decide to dump you. At the very least, poor report card scores could force you to renegotiate a contract or settle for reduced payment. Many experts now claim that costs will ultimately begin to level off. The main differentiator between hospitals will be quality or value. I think the key will be value rather than quality alone.

$$\text{The value equation looks like this: Value} = \frac{\text{Quality}}{\text{Price}}$$

This means that the more you charge, the lower the value you offer your customer. Or, the higher the quality of your care, the higher the value for the purchaser. But what this also means is that higher quality can accommodate higher price and still offer good value. Higher quality can help you strengthen your bottom line.

As a quality measure, patient satisfaction will play a major role. Of course, hard clinical indicators such as morbidity, mortality, length of stay, or infection rates are important indicators of quality. They affect the bottom line of health plans and self-insured employers, and they must be considered. But patients will increasingly vote with their feet, and their vote is based on their own perceptions of quality. If an HMO, employer, or purchasing group has to choose between two hospitals with relatively similar risk-adjusted clinical outcome figures, then patient satisfaction will likely sway the decision. Moreover, lay boards may have little understanding of such indicators as "risk-adjusted length of stay for DRG 237." Everyone understands patient satisfaction, however.

A final note on accountability: Tu and his colleagues (Tu et al. 2001, 1710) warn clinicians to "know your outcomes before others do." This means that ongoing satisfaction monitoring is essential to identifying and addressing internal problems before they show up on external report cards. The jury is still out on how accrediting entities, payers, state hospital associations, and others will use report card data for determining accreditation, reimbursements, etc. There is, as yet, no hard evidence that the general public (i.e., your potential patients) will pay much attention to the data in report cards. Report cards may indeed become more common. But for the foreseeable future, the *quality* part of the value equation will still be driven not by published data but by patients personally experiencing your care, telling others about it, and deciding to use you again. That is serious accountability.

THE LINK TO RISK MANAGEMENT

Adding to the competition for patients and contracts, litigiousness among patients is growing. Malpractice insurers (e.g., St. Paul) are getting out of the business, and premiums are on the rise. The unsettling trend in America to view problems, mistakes, and misfortune as "not my fault" is not limited to healthcare. People do not want to accept the consequences of their own behavior. Still less do they want to accept what they perceive as injury from others.

Healthcare is different from other purchasable goods or services in that its performance affects one's very life. Americans generally have a sensible attitude toward the limits of performance by most types of professionals for hire, but healthcare is something else. Less than perfect performance can mean disability, discomfort, or death. Healthcare had better be perfect! The medical establishment itself has long fostered this myth of medical perfection by refusing to admit the possibility for error or poor judgment. ("They might sue us" is the rationale.) The growth of malpractice claims is the result.

Patients who are more satisfied are less likely to sue—period. All studies of malpractice claims show the same result. Communication is the key to the vast majority of suits. Anger, not injury, is the trigger for most claims. Whether the focus is on hospitals or physicians being sued, conclusions are the same: Empathy and good interpersonal skills prevent malpractice claims (Levinson 1994; Levinson et al. 1997; Krowinski and Steiber 1996; Brown et al. 1993, 13; Mack et al. 1995, 14; Troyer and Salman 1986, 384). Typical of these findings is a study of claims among Florida obstetricians. No relationship was found between prior malpractice claims and present technical quality of the physician. Rather, the authors found that obstetricians who were sued more often also triggered more complaints of poor interpersonal care. These complaints came from all types of patients, not just those who filed claims (Hickson et al. 1994; Entman et al. 1994).

In truth, suing the caregiver, whether physician or hospital, is something patients prefer not to do. Every risk manager knows that less than 3 percent of reported incidents result in claims. They also know that many claims arise from unreported or imagined incidents. This means that there is a huge emotional component to biting the hand that heals you. Anger or frustration, not aggressive lawyers or actual injury, underlie most claims. Even though the average claim never gets to the court stage, it nonetheless costs the provider money via bill write-offs or legal fees.

Elsewhere, I have suggested that dissatisfaction can negatively predispose a patient toward the caregivers (Press 1984). A negative predisposition creates a mind-set that encourages the patient to put a more negative spin on both unusual and normal events. When more satisfied, the patient is positively predisposed toward the caregivers and toward events that occur while under the caregiver's control. The following equations make the point:

1. Higher Patient Satisfaction $=$ Positive Predisposition

2. $\dfrac{\text{Positive}}{\text{Predisposition}} + \dfrac{\text{Negative}}{\text{Incident}} =$ Less Likelihood of Claim

What this adds up to is that patient satisfaction is ultimately the most useful strategy for risk prevention. The cheapest claim to deal with is the one that is prevented because the patient does not think of it or want to do it in the first place.

When Baptist Health Care of Pensacola, Florida, first thought of instituting a serious patient satisfaction program, their scores placed them as low as the 10th percentile among their national peers. By the end of 1995, Baptist had faced 60 malpractice claims and shelled out more than $200,000 in settlements. A vigorous patient satisfaction program was subsequently implemented. By the end of 1997, Baptist ranked in the 98th percentile nationally. In 1998, only 20 malpractice claims were made, with a total payout of $23,000—an almost a tenfold decrease! Only four claims had been made by the end of the third quarter of 1999. Risk management processes themselves had not been altered. The drop in claims was primarily a result of increased patient satisfaction (Taylor 1999, 47). For their efforts, Baptist was MMI Companies' and *Modern Healthcare's* 1999 Excellence in Healthcare Risk Management Award recipient.

CONCLUSIONS

As in many other industries, product and service are indistinguishable in healthcare. Healthcare, after all, is essentially a service industry, with interaction and intervention (as opposed to a tangible object) constituting the product. The manner in which care is delivered has an effect on outcome—both perceived and physically experienced. From diagnosis to medical management, all aspects of care require sensitive interaction between provider and patient. Decor and amenities, attitudes, professional role behavior, content, and mode of information giving—all these factors have an impact on the effectiveness of and the patient's evaluation of care. Thus, the distinction between care and service is moot. All care consists of service as well as technical intervention. Patient satisfaction is another way of referring to the patient's evaluation of care. Patients continually evaluate and reevaluate care as they experience the hospital, clinic, or physician's office. Because this evaluation has an impact on the effectiveness of care both during and after its delivery, patient satisfaction is a component as well as an outcome and measure of care quality.

Because it is a component of care, patient satisfaction affects medical management and thus costs. More satisfied patients will use fewer resources and require less time in treatment. As today's patients are tomorrow's customers, satisfaction also translates into market share. And because your patients are also the customers of health plans, higher satisfaction means stronger competitive position *vis a vis* managed care contracts. Patient satisfaction also translates into job satisfaction for staff, which in turn can result in lower turnover and more effective recruiting. This is particularly important in an era of chronic nursing shortages. Finally, satisfied patients are less likely to seek legal action as the means to resolve negative issues.

What this all adds up to is that patient satisfaction is an inseparable part of care, quality, and successful healthcare operations. Patient satisfaction is a potent mechanism for increasing and sustaining your quality, efficiency, market share, and bottom line. Best of all, efforts to improve patient satisfaction more than pay for themselves. To be a patient satisfaction–driven organization does not take big bucks—only commitment.

ACTION FOR SATISFACTION

1. Educate everyone in your organization about the value of patient satisfaction for their mission and for their job security. The overriding characteristic of a patient satisfaction–driven organization is universal commitment by staff at all levels. Commitment comes when staff, especially top management, believe that high patient satisfaction is essential to achieving the organization's mission. Such an orientation does not automatically come with the territory; if it did, then patient satisfaction would not be an issue today. Education is required. Quite apart from the organizational changes required, staff must be educated in the advantages (for themselves and for their employer) of a patient satisfaction–driven culture. Written material (such as this book) should be distributed to all.

2. Organize discussion groups that ask, "What's in it for me?" Focus on the advantages of a patient satisfaction orientation for each specific department or type of staff. Keep the group size modest to encourage interchange. In the discussion groups, each staff member can be required to share with others an example of how their own jobs could be easier, more rewarding, and more secure if patient satisfaction were high. When a number of people share these personal insights (even if some examples appear rather forced or tenuously linked to patient satisfaction), it is easier for staff to begin buying into the strategy. If each discussion group consisted of representatives from different departments, including different levels of staff, then they might highlight the broad usefulness of patient satisfaction to the overall success of the organization.

REFERENCES

Atkins, P. M., B. S. Marshall, and R. G. Javalgi. 1996. "Happy Employees Lead to Loyal Patients: Survey of Nurses and Patients Shows a Strong Link Between

Employee Satisfaction and Patient Loyalty." *Journal of Healthcare Marketing* 16 (4): 14–23.

Brown, S. W., A. M. Nelson, S. D. Wood, and S. J. Bronkesh. 1993. *Patient Satisfaction Pays: Quality Service for Practice Success*. Gaithersburg, MD: Aspen Publishers, Inc.

Entman, S. S., C. A. Glass, G. B. Hickson, P. B. Githens, K. Whetten-Goldstein, and F. A. Sloan. 1994. "The Relationship Between Malpractice Claims History and Subsequent Obstetric Care." *JAMA* 279: 1588–91.

Garman, A. N., J. Garcia, and M. Hargreaves. 2004. "Patient Satisfaction as a Predictor of Return-to-Provider Behavior: Analysis and Assessment of Financial Implications." *Quality Management in Health Care* 13 (1): 75–80.

Gitomer, J. 1997. "Your Customer's Happiness Requires Partnering Approach." *Business First* 8: 15.

Hibbard, J. H., and J. J. Jewett. 1997. "Will Quality Report Cards Help Consumers?" *Health Affairs* 16 (3): 218–28.

Hickson, G. B., E. W. Clayton, S. S. Entman, C. S. Miller, P. B. Githens, K. Whetten-Goldstein, and F. A. Sloan. 1994. "Obstetricians' Prior Malpractice Experience and Patients' Satisfaction with Care." *JAMA* 272 (20): 1583–87.

Jones, T. O., and W. E. Sasser, Jr. 1995. "Why Satisfied Customers Defect." *Harvard Business Review* 73 (6): 88–102.

Kenagy, J. W., D. M. Berwick, and M. F. Shore. 1999. "Service Quality in Health Care." *JAMA* 281 (7): 661–65.

Kenkel, P. J. 1995. *Report Cards: What Every Health Provider Needs to Know About HEDIS and Other Performance Measures*. Gaithersburg. MD: Aspen Publishers, Inc.

Krowinski, W. J., and S. R. Steiber. 1996. *Measuring and Managing Patient Satisfaction*, 2nd ed. Chicago: American Hospital Publishing, Inc.

Kurata, J. H., A. N. Nogawa, D. M. Phillips, S. Hoffman, and M. N. Werblun. 1992. "Patient and Provider Satisfaction with Medical Care." *Journal of Family Practice* 35 (2): 176–79.

Levinson, W. 1994. "Physician-Patient Communication: A Key to Malpractice Prevention." *JAMA* 272 (20): 1619–20.

Levinson, W., D. L. Roter, J. P. Mullooly, V. T. Dull, and R. M. Frankel. 1997. "Physician-Patient Communication: The Relationship with Malpractice Claims Among Primary Care Physicians and Surgeons." *JAMA* 277 (7): 553–59.

Mack, J. L., K. M. File, J. E. Horwitz, and R. A. Prince. 1995. "The Effect of Urgency on Patient Satisfaction and Future Emergency Department Choice." *Healthcare Management Review* 20 (2): 7–15.

Mayer, T., and R. Cates. 2004. *Leadership for Great Customer Services: Satisfied Patients, Satisfied Employees.* Chicago: Health Administration Press.

Moran, N. Y., and M. P. Malone. 1997. "Utilizing Patient Satisfaction to Meet the Challenges of Managed Health Care." *Home Health Outcomes and Resource Utilization: Integrating Today's Critical Priorities,* edited by C. E. Adams and A. Anthony, 63–77. New York: National League for Nursing Press.

Nelson, E. C., R. T. Rust, A. Zahorik, R. L. Rose, P. Batalden, and B. A. Siemanski. 1992. "Do Patient Perceptions of Quality Relate to Hospital Financial Performance?" *Journal of Health Care Marketing* 12 (4): 6–13.

Oliver, R. L. 1996. *Satisfaction: A Behavioral Perspective on the Consumer.* New York: McGraw-Hill.

Press Ganey Associates. 2005. "Physician and Patient Satisfaction." Unpublished research report.

————. 2002. "Patient Satisfaction and Hospital Profitability: A National Study." Internal research report.

————. 1998. "Present Profit and Past Satisfaction." Unpublished research report.

Press, I. 1984. "The Predisposition to File Claims: The Patient's Perspective." *Law, Medicine and Health Care* 12 (2): 53–61.

Schlesinger, L. A., and J. L. Heskett. 1991. "Customer Satisfaction Is Rooted in Employee Satisfaction." *Harvard Business Review* (Nov/Dec): 148–49.

Strasser, S., and R. M. Davis. 1991. *Measuring Patient Satisfaction for Improved Patient Services.* Chicago: Health Administration Press.

Taylor, M. 1999. "Paying Attention to the Healthcare Customer." *Modern Healthcare,* October 25, 47–48.

Technical Assistance Research Programs, Inc. (TARP). 1976. *Consumer Complaint Handling in America: Final Report.* Washington, DC: Office of Consumer Affairs.

Troyer, G. T., and S. L. Salman (eds). 1986. *Handbook of Health Care Risk Management.* Rockville, MD: Aspen Systems, Corp.

Tu, J. V., M. J. Schull, L. E. Ferris, J. E. Hux, and D. A. Redelmeier. 2001. "Problems for Clinical Judgement: 4. Surviving in the Report Card Era." *Canadian Medical Association Journal* 164 (12): 1709–12.

Tumlinson, A., H. Bottigheimer, P. Mahoney, E. M. Stone, and A. Hendricks. 1997. "Choosing a Health Plan: What Information Will Consumers Use?" *Health Affairs* 16 (3): 229–38.

Ware, J. E. Jr., and A. R. Davies. 1984. "Behavioral Consequences of Consumer

Dissatisfaction with Medical Care." *Evaluation and Program Planning* 6 (3–4): 291–97.

Wolosin, R. J. 2004. "What Do Doctors Want? Press Ganey Physician Satisfaction Services." *Satisfaction Monitor* (July/Aug): 4–7.

Zimmerman, D., and J. J. Skalko. 1994. *Reengineering Health Care: A Vision for the Future*. Franklin, WI: Eagle Press.

CHAPTER 3

The Basics of Patient Satisfaction

PATIENT SATISFACTION IS a summation of all the patient's experiences in the hospital. Satisfaction can be high or low. When we talk of increasing or improving patient satisfaction, we are talking about enhancing the experience of care, resulting in a more positive patient evaluation.

WHAT IS BEING EVALUATED?

As suggested earlier, for patients, "service" translates into "care," and service consists of many different types of interactions and experiences.

Customer service circles speak of "moments of truth." In healthcare, these moments essentially refer to any experiences that can have an effect on the patient's predisposition toward the caregiver. The experiences can be mundane, positive, or terrifying: a dirty floor, a surprisingly tasty dessert, a receptionist who talks on the phone and is oblivious to the patient standing next to the desk, a physician leaving the room before the patient fully understands the explanation or instructions, empathy and clear explanations from the nurse as she inserts a catheter, or an unkept promise that the doctor would be back in ten minutes.

Imagine the hundreds of sights, sounds, impressions, events, and interactions that every patient experiences in your hospital— from the first glimpse of your sign and the entrance to the parking lot to the functioning of the lobby door at the moment of discharge. Actually, the patient's experience often begins even earlier, with the physician practice (that you may own or with which you contract) or in the outpatient clinic, lab, or radiology department of the hospital where preadmission testing is done.

All interactions and experiences in the hospital are potential moments of truth. The patient does not recognize a meaningful distinction between technical and interpersonal experiences. To complicate matters, the number of experiences that form an evaluation could almost be doubled because experiences of family and friends affect the patient's overall evaluation of the institution and the care. Patient satisfaction is most often a result of consensus rather than a solitary evaluation by the patient alone. Spouses and children can have significant input to the patient's evaluation of care. Indeed, in many instances the spouse or mature child fills out the patient satisfaction survey. As the baby boomers age, this second-hand evaluating is going to happen more frequently.

An experience becomes a moment of truth if it is particularly positive or negative and thereby makes an impression. The incoming patient and her husband ask a housekeeping employee directions to the nursing unit and are escorted in person. The patient and spouse are positively affected. The obstetrician resident in Labor and Delivery repeatedly passes the bed of the young, single mother-to-be and never stops to give a few friendly words of encouragement or to reassuringly squeeze her foot. The mother does not consciously expect a foot squeeze, so she does not really note its absence, but an opportunity for a positive moment of truth has been missed. Again, any act of omission or commission can affect patient perceptions. Singly in some cases and collectively in others, these acts can have a significant impact on the patient's overall evaluation of and (as we noted earlier) response to care.

Because any experience could have a conscious effect on the patient, producing a definitive list of all potential moments of truth is impossible—let alone coming up with suggestions for making a positive experience of each moment. Moreover, not all hospital experiences are equal. A dirty floor, poor signage, or cold soup can affect patient satisfaction with the overall hospital experience, but these are not the same as a painful IV start or poor information about a scary-sounding test. Nor do these details have the same effect on patients as does staff inattention to the social and emotional experience of sickness and hospitalization.

In general, the following rank order holds for the inpatient experience.

1. Good food counts more than lousy food.
2. Friendliness counts more than good food.
3. Communication counts more than friendliness when information exchange is necessary.
4. Empathy enhances communication.

Analogous elements hold for emergency, outpatient, and all other patient contacts within the clinical setting. The comfort and cleanliness of the emergency waiting room are more significant than food. Friendliness is always important. Communication is always important, and empathy makes communication more effective. In the ED, waiting time becomes an important issue, but (as we shall discuss later) good communication—explanations for delays—can significantly mitigate the effect of waiting time.

Notice that technical quality is not mentioned in the hierarchy above. That is because it is assumed. IV drip rates, appropriateness of medications, appropriateness of surgical technique used—all are issues of technical quality that patients typically do not perceive or evaluate. Ask anyone what he or she wants of a visit to the doctor or hospital and you will get a pretty consistent answer: "competent diagnosis and/or cure." If asked whether they would forgo this for friendliness, communication and empathy, most would give a resounding, "No!" This being said, we must emphasize once again that patients *do* judge your technical quality but base their perceptions on interactions and experiences that could be described as service issues. These issues are encompassed in the list above.

Of course, this hierarchical list is simplistic. Communication is important, but what should be communicated? What should staff empathize with? Even "good food" is not a simple issue. Does a Cambodian or Japanese migrant feel comfortable eating a high-quality, "standard" American breakfast of eggs, hot cakes, sausages, and coffee? Good food is not necessarily *appropriate* food. Will a rural Mexican migrant with severe dehydration and diarrhea (a cold disease) feel confident about the sensitivity and quality of care if orange juice (a cold food) is offered with a meal? From this patient's experience, everyone should know that cold foods can make cold diseases worse; only opposites can cure![1]

All of this suggests that patient satisfaction is far more complex than is commonly assumed.

EXPECTATIONS AND HOPES

We must be realistic. Patients do not have expectations about all aspects of clinical care. Some patients have past experience with the acute care setting, while others have none. Even those with prior clinical experience may not be in the hospital for the same procedures and interactions with the same types of staff. Thus, no patient comes to the clinical encounter with a complete set of clear expectations about care. First-timers may bring few specific expectations to the hospital. They may expect that registration will be efficient and easy, but they will probably have no preconceived idea about what occurs during registration or why certain questions are asked. Patients may know what an IV is but, beyond hoping that it will be relatively painless, may have little idea of who usually does it, precisely where the needle is inserted, or what the drip rate indicates.

I remember the first time I had an IV. First, I was appalled and sickened by the needle being inserted into the back of my hand. That is not a natural place to stick a needle! What if I moved my hand, and the needle wiggled about? It would pierce the vein, and I would bleed to death! Later, the fluid in the clear plastic bag was running out. I had seen enough B movies and TV whodunnits to know that you can kill someone by injecting air into a vein. I pounded the call button vigorously. The nurse took forever to answer the call (almost five minutes—an eternity when death is so imminent!). She informed me that the machine next to the bed, the drip-regulating mechanism, prevents any air from getting into the vein and that the IV would be automatically shut down if the fluid ran out. The information calmed me, but not before I had spent those terrifying minutes with my ignorance. I also felt somewhat embarrassed. After all, I was a college professor and should have known about the IV. I felt that I had made a fool of myself. I also felt that I had been taken for granted, and that is not very satisfying. Afterwards, if I had gotten a patient survey in the mail, I would have rated the technical quality of the IV as no more than a three on a five-point scale. I have subsequently had several other IVs and can say that, in retrospect, that first stick was probably closer to a five in technical competence. But this is immaterial, because I had already complained to family and friends about that first IV.

I had come to the hospital with no IV experience—or clear expectations about IVs—yet I felt quite capable of evaluating it both during and afterward. Having no prior experience with clinical care does not mean the patient lacks a basis for evaluating it. Each event stimulates an evaluation by the patient.

Expectations are assumptions of performance. They are based on:

- past clinical experiences of self and significant others;

- logic— "It should be done this way"—which is also informed by family, community, and cultural values; and
- custom—"It's usually done this way."

In other words, expectations are essentially evidence based. A patient's expectation about care suggests an element of control (e.g., "At least you know what to expect"), even if the expectation is negative (e.g., "The cortisone shot will probably hurt"). Because expectations anticipate a certain level of performance quality, merely meeting a positive expectation will not ordinarily result in the highest patient satisfaction. If you expect empathetic, skilled, knowledgeable, informative nursing—and get it—then you will be satisfied but not necessarily wowed. You will think, "It's what should have happened in the first place." When expectations of any kind are met—no matter how positive they are—the result is no surprise; the care is appropriate but not special.

Expectations, of course, can be positive or negative. If you expect the hospital food to be lousy—and it is—then you will not be satisfied. This is why asking survey questions about whether expectations were met does not work. Assume on a survey you are asked how well nursing met your expectations and how well the food service met your expectations. Assume you expected great nursing and lousy food. Assume you got both. You would give both issues high marks for meeting your expectations!

Any expectation—even a negative one—is useful in that by simply thinking you know what to expect, even if it is pain, uncertainty is minimized and stress can be anticipated and controlled. However, meeting negative expectations does not mean you are satisfying your patients. Things may be more predictable, but certainly not more pleasant.

Meeting or surpassing different kinds of expectations can have different implications:

- Positive performance expectations met = satisfaction
- Positive expectations surpassed = higher satisfaction
- Negative expectations met = dissatisfaction

- Negative expectations surpassed = satisfaction to highest satisfaction

When negative expectations are surpassed, patients are being positively surprised or delighted. Negative expectations are always accompanied by hopes. Hopes are wishes, not anticipations of performance. You do not expect them to be met. Hopes differ significantly from expectations in that hopes are based on a lack of knowledge and reflect fear and uncertainty.

For example, you are led to a treatment cubicle in the ED; you expect a delay because you have heard many horror stories about EDs, but you hope the doctor will come in quickly. In another instance, you come in for your first cortisone shot in your elbow; you expect it will hurt but hope it won't. You expect mediocre hospital food; you hope it will be acceptable, but you do not even hope for delicious. On the other hand, you expect competent, empathetic nurses. No hopeful thinking is involved here—the nurses had better be good.

For many of the experiences and events they will encounter, patients (particularly first-timers) have no clear expectations—only hopes—that

- staff will be competent;
- treatment will be fast;
- treatment will not be uncomfortable;
- treatment will be effective;
- the patient will be out quickly; and
- the patient will feel better.

Hopes tend to be more idealized and simplistic than expectations, and they are quite often unachievable. However, because hopes are idealized, satisfaction is automatically high when hopes are realized.

Thus, clinical staff must have some idea about patients' expectations and hopes regarding their clinical experiences. Expectations are more specific than hopes. To at least some extent, they are based on past healthcare experiences (of the patient or others) and logic (e.g., rational business practices, consumer orientation). Ostensibly, therefore, hospitals should find it easier to meet expectations than hopes. When you know patients' expectations, you are in a better position to modify your technical, informational, or organizational performance. Expectations may also require special explanations to foster a more realistic understanding of the limitations of clinical care.

Hopes, on the other hand, being idealized and general, require reassurance, support, and empathy as well as explanations about anticipated aspects of care. Providing what the patient hopes for may be impossible. Recovery from knee surgery is never painless, despite a patient's hopes. So long as the patient knows that your intentions are to realize what they hope for, but that the realization of the hope may be thwarted by the limitations of medicine or hospital organization (not your personal limitations—that only creates dissatisfaction with the quality of the staff!), patients will be forgiving and understanding. And they will be satisfied with the care they do receive.

Staff should elicit patient expectations and hopes prior to any procedures, prognoses, or discussions of disease management. By knowing what patients expect or hope, you can deal with erroneous conceptions or clarify your limitations before a perfectly normal but unsatisfactory experience occurs.

SATISFACTION AS A PRODUCT OF INTERACTION BETWEEN TWO CULTURES

Patient satisfaction is a product of what both participants—the patient and the caregiver—bring to the clinical encounter. Patient satisfaction is not a one-sided product of the hospital and its staff, of proper clinical procedures, and of basic courtesy. Patient perceptions of care are always filtered through a cloak of culture, experiences, hopes, and expectations. Thus, although communication and empathy are important, what to communicate and empathize with is not necessarily obvious or common sense. Patients, not clinical staff, define the content and performance criteria for satisfying care. Staff must understand something about the patient if satisfaction is to progress beyond a basic level of experience with simple service factors such as food, housekeeping, decor, and common courtesy.

Patients' primary needs are broad based and certainly not merely service focused. These needs include accurate diagnosis; information about the condition, procedures, and prognosis; comfort during and after the procedure (be it medical or surgical); clear, realistic discharge instructions; and, last but most important, cure—if not cure, then at least some hope. Patients want to be taken seriously both as patients and as real people whose family and social and economic lives have been threatened or disrupted by the medical problem and by the isolation and disorientation of hospitalization. Smiles, eye contact, courtesy, and ethnically sensitive food may help, but they are not the primary reason for the patient's presence in your stress-inducing institution. Remember, all things being equal, patients would rather not use your services! More preferable places exist for nice decor, smiling folks, and good chow.

To achieve sustained, exceptional patient satisfaction, go beyond the generic service issues. Understand that the interaction between our medical system and the patient is an interaction of cultures, each of which is incompletely known to the other.

Certainly, patients in an industrialized society are part of the wider culture. They are committed to modern medicine—both official and popular. In medical anthropology, we refer to our modern medical system as a closed system. This means that in our system, body and self are largely unrelated; health is independent of the patient's moral, social, religious, and economic life. That is, sickness is not a punishment but a naturally occurring mechanical event. Lifestyle may affect susceptibility but does not directly cause most diseases. You do not get a venereal disease because you have sinned, but rather because you contracted a virus. Gall stones, prostate cancer, heart attack, or phlebitis are impersonal diseases, largely unrelated to the patient's identity, reputation, and behavior toward others. One's religious, economic, family, social, or political behavior is not a sufficient cause of disease. Our medical system is amoral, impersonal, and mechanical. Cure is also impersonal, mechanical, and universal. *Universal* refers to the fact that a particular disease (e.g., syphilis) has the same cause and cure for all patients, regardless of who they are.

The average patient's medical system, on the other hand, is open. To most of us, sickness is never an impersonal, anonymous event. Body and self are closely allied. Disease threatens one's identity and economic and social obligations (perhaps one's very existence), and its effect is always personal and always has implications for all other aspects of the individual's life. Every instance of sickness calls our strength, competence, and attractiveness into question. These beliefs and feelings can have a significant effect on the patient's expectations of and response to care.

In addition to anxieties and threats to roles and identities, patients bring a complex baggage of beliefs about health and sickness, expectations about healing and healers, and misconceptions about hospitals and treatment to the clinical encounter. The encounter is further complicated by its occurring in a strange, unintelligible, uncontrollable context—the hospital, physician's office, or clinic.

All of this constitutes patient culture, and it is brought by every patient to the hospital or physician's office.

It would be easy at this point to summarize by saying that clinicians must know something about patient culture to maximize satisfaction and the quality of care, but it is not that simple. If patients' personal beliefs, anxieties, and expectations can influence their experience and evaluation of care, then so too can clinical culture influence that experience. An understanding of where the patient is coming from is insufficient if this knowledge is filtered through a clinical culture that that does not know where *it* is coming from. A lack of self-knowledge impedes accommodation of the patients' needs. If patients' beliefs, expectations, anxieties, and personal issues are understood yet viewed by staff as illegitimate, erroneous, or irrelevant, then the result will be missed opportunities for reassurance and optimization of care. To satisfy patients, you must know something about yourself as well as them.

Thus, it is imperative that staff recognize their own culture. Clinicians bring an equally complex baggage of beliefs, expectations, misconceptions, family roles, prejudices, professional and personal identities, organizational culture, and hospital roles to the encounter with patients. Staff professional values, for example, can lead to lack of respect for patients' presenting complaints. Harried ED staff may roll their eyes when a parent with a snively nosed kid demands immediate attention. Here, a professional trained to deal with major trauma could feel abused by patients who present with "inappropriate" complaints. Such values, prejudices, or whatever you might call them might be expressed behaviorally through do-the-minimum examination and interaction that are adequate—but no more than that. This attitude can be sensed by the patient.

Organizational rules can also affect staff sensitivity to patient needs. For example, documentation is essential for many reasons: to create continuity of care from shift to shift, to coordinate among different staff and specialties, to meet external regulatory requirements, to establish a paper trail for risk management, and so forth. Regardless of their functionality, paperwork requirements can result in slower staff response to patients. No matter how firmly we argue that paperwork is a necessary part of care, patients do not see it this way. Paperwork is not the hands-on care that patients want or that they base their evaluations on. It appears to be an optional, ostensibly postponable activity that takes staff time away from direct patient care. In other words, paperwork is a part of hospital culture (and thus amenable to modification), not part of the technical act of healing.

CONCLUSIONS

All things being equal, patients never, ever want to use your services.[2] When they do enter your hospital, they are not there for the food, decor, or company. They are there for the serious business of diagnosis and/or cure. Patients' familiar routines, timetables, and social and economic identities, if not their very lives, are threatened by the sickness and hospitalization. Under these circumstances, any event or interaction, including the surroundings and machinery, experienced while under the hospital's care may significantly influence the patient's response to and evaluation of that care.

Of course, typical service issues (e.g., friendliness, timeliness, surroundings) are important because they are among the most familiar and intelligible things the patient experiences in the hospital. These services are necessary but insufficient for high patient satisfaction. Patient and hospital represent two very different cultures. To achieve high levels of patient satisfaction, hospitals must progress beyond these low-hanging fruit to learn more about both patients and themselves. Each represents a culture with its own values, expectations, and behaviors. Clinical staff must learn more about the effect of sickness and hospitalization upon patients' personal lives and their experiences of healthcare. At the same time, staff must learn more about their own culture—the personal and professional rules, values, and habits that affect their evaluation of and response to patients.

ACTION FOR SATISFACTION

1. Assume the following:
   - The patient is a stranger in a strange place.
   - Patients know nothing about the hospital and its rituals and routines.

- Patients will easily misinterpret what you are doing or saying.
- Patients are constantly judging your hospital and the performance of every individual with whom they come in contact.
- Every experience has some effect on the patient's evaluation of care.

2. Work with staff at all levels to develop an orientation toward patient satisfaction. So many things happen to the patient that it is impossible to specify appropriate tactics for dealing with individuals in specific situations. Familiarize staff with the five assumptions above and initiate discussion about how best to respond to each.

3. Encourage staff from the CEO down to develop an orientation that views the hospital as their home and the patients as guests. Would you be continually friendly toward houseguests in spite of your own worries or stresses? Would a guest be left wandering in a hallway without someone asking if help or information is needed? Would you pass by a gum wrapper on the floor of your home without picking it up? Would you serve a meal and not ask if there were something else the guest might want? Would you barge into the guest's room without knocking? The guest/home orientation is a general one that, if actively exhibited and rewarded by administration, will cover a myriad of situations—including unpredictable ones.

4. Second-guess your patients. Assume they know nothing about what is being done, yet they want to. Staff must be encouraged to imagine questions that patients might have about procedures and events, and discuss explanations that could answer these questions—ideally before the questions are asked. Assume patients have expectations about care that differ from yours and that your motives and actions will be misinterpreted. With the guest/home model and with the significance of information and explanation in mind, the

opportunity exists to create and exceed expectations during the patient's stay.

5. Elicit patients' expectations and hopes about their treatment. Devise strategies to meet the expectations or explain why they cannot be met.

6. Examine your own culture for roadblocks to sensitive care. Have staff identify rules and regulations that could affect patients receiving timely, efficient, sensitive care. Start by asking staff to identify really stupid rules.[3] This is fun and focuses analytical attention on the often arbitrary nature of regulations. Then, expand the focus to rules that are logical yet may be nonetheless arbitrary. For example, some hospitals require that only nurses be permitted to pass meal trays. The rationale is that only nurses know what patients should or should not be eating, and that if food service staff were allowed to pass trays, then serious health-endangering errors could result.

   Given that many hospitals allow food service staff to pass trays without endangering patients, a good discussion could result in reevaluation of rules that impede timely service. A similar rationale lies behind a common rule that only nurses be allowed to respond to patient call buttons. Some hospitals require that the staff member closest to the patient's room, regardless of that person's job in the hospital, respond to the call. A nurse is notified, if required. Often the patient wants some service that anyone could provide, and this saves time for busy nurses. Discussions about such rules can lead to increased sensitivity toward hospital practices that often result from turf protection rather than sound patient care needs.

7. Organize workshops in which staff examine their attitudes toward patients. Attempt to identify categories of problem patients (e.g., by payer, by ethnicity and race, by type of medical problem or procedure, by personality characteristics). Are these feelings based on stereotypes or consistent experiences with these types of patients? Discuss why such attitudes exist and what their potential effect could be on style of interaction

with patients and on medical management decisions. How can such attitudes be modified while at the same time recognizing that some types of patients do indeed cause emotional or organizational problems for staff?

NOTES

1. In many rural areas of Mexico, ancient humoral medicine beliefs are still strong. Foods, diseases, and medicines are defined as either hot or cold—categories having nothing to do with actual temperature. Opposites cure, so if one suffers from a cold disease, then a hot medicinal is required. Penicillin, for example, is cold. An anthropologist colleague of mine tells of Mexican patients in a Texas hospital who refused to take penicillin for diarrhea, but found it acceptable if mixed with chocolate (a hot substance), which combated the coldness of the penicillin.

2. An exception may be childbirth. After the birth, and particularly if the new mother stays for several days, the woman is far more a customer than a patient. For some women, a day or two in the hospital is a time for being pampered and a time to gather courage before plunging into the responsibilities of childcare at home without skilled nurses and physicians hanging about.

Childbirth is ostensibly a happy, celebratory occasion. The more memorable a hospital can make the experience, the more likely the mother is to think of returning when and if some future medical need arises. The maternity unit offers a prime marketing opportunity for the hospital.

3. The Disney Institute uses the terms *red rules* and *blue rules*. Red rules can never be broken, and there are not many—no smoking around oxygen, for example. Blue rules are hospital operational rules and can be changed.

CHAPTER 4

Digging Deeper:
Patient Versus Clinical Cultures

PATIENT SATISFACTION DERIVES from the patient's evaluation of how well the provider meets his or her personal and emotional as well as physical needs.

Sending your staff to smile school will have only a modest effect on your patients' satisfaction. Patients bring a complex cultural baggage to the clinical encounter. Our closed medical system, as defined in the last chapter, does not typically recognize other parts of the culture as direct causes or symptoms of sickness. Indeed, clinicians can easily minimize such cultural manifestations as noise.

Patients, on the other hand, work with an eclectic, open system of medicine. Although U.S. patients typically believe in modern medicine and its impersonal, mechanical paradigm of causality and cure, the effect of disease on a patient is anything but impersonal and mechanical. Roles and identities are threatened. Moreover, as disease disrupts lives and lifestyles—or, at the very least, our daily plans—patients have coping mechanisms for dealing with symptoms, sickness, and disability. In other words, all patients come to the hospital with their own medical systems. Those who work in the clinical setting should have some idea of the complexity of this system, because true patient satisfaction derives from the interaction of patient culture and clinical culture.

At first, the discussion that follows might seem more appropriate for physicians than for others in the clinical setting—but this is not so. Patients' medical beliefs, habits, and personal histories can affect all interactions with all staff, and they certainly have an impact on compliance after discharge. Given that dietary or housekeeping personnel—let alone nurses, technologists, and therapists—have more contact with the patient than the doctor does, the job of understanding where the patient's coming from belongs to everyone.

ILLNESS VERSUS DISEASE

Medical anthropologists, who study the cultural components of sickness and healing, find it extremely helpful to conceptualize the difference between medical and patient cultures as a difference between illness and disease (e.g., Kleinman Eisenberg, and Good 1978).

Disease can be defined as biomedicine's definition of sickness and the physical impact and manifestation of sickness. *Illness* can be defined as the patient's definition and view of sickness and the social and emotional effect and manifestations of sickness.

Here, "sickness" is the neutral term. Because patients always have some ideas about their physical problem, and because there are always emotional and social costs to being sick, every case of disease is typically accompanied by an illness. Disease and illness may vary independently. As the patient is treated, effects of the disease may dwindle. At the same time, anxiety about the disease, missed work, unkept obligations, future health, and so forth may increase. These concerns form part of the illness. The illness includes all of the effects of the sickness, not just those that are physically sensed. Illness may thus exist in the absence of disease. Illness is always personal. Its effects happen to you and threaten your self-image and identity—whether that is as a superwoman, provider, spouse, professional, or dependable friend.

A large part of patient satisfaction results from the hospital and its staff addressing the patient's illness as well as the disease. A dramatic gap can exist between the two. "To state it flatly," says Eisenberg (1977, 11), "patients suffer 'illnesses'; physicians diagnose and treat 'diseases'." By recognizing and responding to the illness, providers can go beyond the usual service issues to significantly enhance the patient's experience of care.

EVOLUTION OF AN ILLNESS

An in-depth analysis of the evolution of an illness might help to clarify the concept. The interaction with the physician or the treatment in the hospital is merely the last phase of a highly complex process.

Symptoms

Illness begins with the sensation of symptoms. What is a symptom? Not every sensation of pain or discomfort is necessarily defined as a symptom. I ask students in my clinical anthropology class if any of them has experienced pain or discomfort in the previous several days. Over half raise their hands. One says she had a bad headache that morning. Why didn't she go to the student health service? "Because I was out partying last night, and it's just a hangover." Another says he has pain in his left lower back. Why not see a doctor? "Because I was playing basketball yesterday, and I'm just stiff. It'll be okay." Perhaps the kid really is merely stiff, as he suggests, or perhaps he has a major kidney problem. Perhaps the young lady has a tumor. The point is that neither of them interpreted the discomfort as a symptom worth worrying about or worth bringing to the attention of a professional.

We constantly sift symptoms, ignoring or downplaying some and paying attention to others. Each of us has a pain or other odd sensation daily. We ignore it or pop an aspirin and forget it. Studies have indicated that blue collar workers tend to ignore joint and muscle pains: They are just part of the job.

Pain has a large cultural component. Most humans, regardless of race or ethnicity, have pretty similar pain sensitivities. Notice I did not say "pain thresholds" or "tolerances"—that is where culture comes in. Studies indicate that people can take more pain when in the company of their significant others. Pain experienced and tolerated during a tough basketball game with one's buddies might cause a disabling and illness-identifying response if the same level of pain occurs when one is alone. Suggestion can also affect pain tolerance. In a fascinating study of pain, Lambert, Libman, and Poser (1960) selected a panel of Protestant and Jewish students at a large university. Individually and in private, they tested the pain tolerance of each student and found few differences. After establishing baseline tolerances for each student, they then told half the Protestant subjects (again, individually and in private) that Jewish kids could take more pain than Protestants. The other half they told that Jewish kids could take less pain. They did the same with the Jewish students, telling half that Protestants can take more pain and half that Protestants can take less than Jews. Then they retested all the students, again in private. Both groups of Protestant students increased their pain tolerance. The Jewish group that was told they could take less pain than Protestants also increased their pain tolerance. But the Jews who were told they could take more pain than Protestants stayed relatively stable in pain tolerance. Apparently, they did not want to appear different.

Pain tolerance is but one culturally mediated aspect of pain. Expression of pain is another. Zborowski's (1952) classic study of Italian, Jewish, and old-American patients is a great example. In his study, he found that Italian and Jewish patients complained more to nurses about pain. The old Americans, defined as third-generation Anglo-Protestants, complained far less. He concluded that to Italians and Jews, sickness was the cue for a social drama. Complaining about pain was expected in their cultures and was rewarded by nurturant behavior. For the old Americans, sickness was something private and reflective of personal weakness. By minimizing complaints, they felt they were calling less attention to their lessened state.

I came across a clear example of culturally mediated pain expression during my year as a visiting professor at a medical school hospital in a culturally heterogeneous city. The obstetric ward there was an ethnic boiling pot. Women of each group expressed pain differently during labor. I noticed that Cuban women tended to complain more when their husbands were within hearing distance. The noise diminished significantly when only their mothers were present. I remember one young Anglo resident who got quite upset at a Cuban woman in labor, who made a lot of noise while her husband lingered visibly at the doorway. The resident yelled at her, telling her not to be "such a baby." When the husband left, the woman quieted down.

Here, the Cuban woman's expressions of pain served an important purpose. In a male-dominated culture, childbirth is one of the few areas controlled by the female. By expressing pain, the woman appears to be both victim and hero to her husband. The medical resident's insensitivity to this (as well as the nurses' and doctors' resentment of the complaining Jewish and Italian patients in the previous example) tells patients that the staff does not really care. The staff, for their part, tend to have their own expectations of what constitutes an appropriate amount of pain expression for any given condition. Too much complaint can be disruptive—it becomes noise and can be resented. Patients can sense this resentment. They can be made to feel that they are doing something wrong. This is dissatisfying.

Validating Symptoms

For some patients, being sick means that certain symptoms should be present. For example, French patients typically believe the liver to be a major locus of health and disease. Being sick means something is wrong with the liver. Thus, a French patient who is ill will likely complain of liver problems in addition to any other symptoms that may be felt. When I was working with patients in Bogota, Colombia, almost every hospitalized patient complained about "pain in the mouth of the stomach" in addition to any other symptoms. Such pains constitute a common validating symptom in Colombian culture. If you complain of pain in the mouth of the stomach, then it validates for others that you are really sick.

In a fascinating study of such validating symptoms, Zola (1966) focused on Italian and Irish patients at an eye clinic. Although they came largely for eye problems, Irish patients tended to complain of discomfort in their nose and throat areas as well. Italians, on the other hand, even when they had an eye or ear disorder, "did not locate their chief complaints there, nor did they focus their future concern on these locations" (628). Here, again, each ethnic group expresses illness through special reference to culturally determined parts of the body—not necessarily those parts that reflect the presenting complaint.

I observed a great example while doing research in a large U.S. urban outpatient clinic.

> *A little old Jewish lady came in to the young resident's office . . .*
>
> Doctor: "How are you doing, Mrs. Goldstein? What's the problem?"
>
> Patient: "Doctor, I'm veak 'n dizzy, I have a svelling in the leg and a pain in the enkle."
>
> Doctor: "How long have you had this swelling, Mrs. Goldstein?"
>
> He asked her a few more questions about the leg, examined her, and determined that she was probably suffering from phlebitis. He wrote a prescription and sent her off.
>
> Afterwards, I asked him if he recalled exactly what Mrs. Goldstein had said as she presented her symptoms. "Sure," he replied. "She said she had a pain and 'svelling' in the leg."

"No," I corrected. "She started out by saying she was 'veak and dizzy.'"

"Oh, yeah, 'veak and dizzy.' They all say that! We call that 'old Jewish people's VD.' We ignore it."

"Veak and dizzy" were Mrs. Goldstein's validating symptoms. It confirmed to her and to her significant others—validating symptoms are as much for others as for oneself—that she was really sick. Here, in dismissing her "VD," the physician ignored the very first of his patient's presenting symptoms. Whether the woman really felt weak and dizzy does not matter. By ignoring that symptom, he told the patient that the doctor does not care.

Explanatory Models

A key component of all illness is the explanatory model, or EM (see Kleinman 1987 for a thorough discussion). The EM is the patient's explanation for what is going on and includes answers to questions such as

- What do I have?
- What caused it?
- Why me?
- What should be done?
- What will happen if it does not get better?

All people everywhere have explanatory models for illness. After all, illness (which patients define as including both accidents and sickness) is the ultimate cause of death. Illness can maim, disable, distress, inconvenience, or kill; thus, illness threatens everyone. All societies have created medical systems to cope with illness, and explanatory models are central to all medical systems. EMs give meaning to the threatening and potentially terrifying state of being sick. EMs help people organize and manage illness by naming the problem and listing the proper course of action. When an illness has been identified and named, it becomes less intangible and frightening. Resources (both medical and personal) can be mobilized. The illness becomes treatable.

The biomedical accuracy of explanatory models is irrelevant. They are logical to the patient. EMs reflect the patient's everyday experiences. They reflect the meaning of life, health, and misfortune to the patient and his or her family and social network. For example, a white, elderly patient believes that behavioral excesses can cause illness. Liquids too hot or too cold, too much emotion, running or moving too fast—all are bad for a person. She was raised in a neighborhood where her immigrant family were the only members of their ethnic group. Sensitive to instances of ethnic prejudice and desirous of blending into America, the patient's mother insisted that excess of any kind called attention to the family and to their ethnic identity. She was fearful of neighbors pointing to "those kids" who ran too fast, hollered too much, or stood out in any way. "Blend in," she would admonish. "This is America." To this immigrant mother—and to the 100 percent American children she raised—excess was the cause of all things dangerous. That excess should also cause illness is but a logical extension.

Explanatory models are not merely medical curiosities or funky objects for study by anthropologists. As with every other part of an illness, EMs can affect medical management and outcomes. The belief (mentioned earlier in our discussion of symptoms) that a pain in the lower left back is stiffness from working out too hard reflects the individual's EM. More than being a cute example of culture at work, this explanatory model can keep the sufferer from seeking timely medical care. A study of white, middle-class, New York male hypertension patients revealed them to have a common explanatory model that classified nervousness and irritability as symptoms of hypertension (Cohen 1979). These patients' EM further embraced the view that when they subsequently felt calm and in control of themselves, their blood pressure was back to normal. Patients with this EM were more likely to become noncompliant by stopping their medications, thus affecting outcome.

The 45-year-old white, middle-class professional man came to the physician practice owned by the hospital that his HMO contracts with complaining of a pain in the calf and swelling in his ankle. The doctor tentatively diagnoses phlebitis. The patient more tentatively offers his explanatory model. Being athletic and a regular squash player, he figures his veins are more efficient than those of a less active man. Having larger veins means slower blood flow—in his logic, fluid flows faster through more constricted pipes than through wider pipes. Slower flowing blood is more likely to form a clot than swifter flowing blood. The physician quickly dismisses this EM and attempts to focus the patient's attention on the real causes of blood clots and the potential danger a clot can pose. Here, the doctor's EM stresses pathology and the debilitating nature of the problem, while the patient's EM stresses the problem's origin in a robust lifestyle and in being too much of a jock. The phlebitis ("an old person's disease," he comments) threatens the patient and his self-image. His EM helps ameliorate the threatening implications. The doctor sees no point in even negotiating an EM.

Here, the patient is left with diminished self-esteem and diminished ownership of the illness. Some trust is lost. The patient may no longer be an active collaborator in treatment.

Explanatory models can range from the mundane (e.g., feed a cold, starve a fever) to the exotic (e.g., witchcraft). Kleinman (1980) notes that the ethnic Chinese EM for mental illness involves a perception that mental illness is a condition that disgraces both the sufferer and his or her family. This EM causes many Chinese who suffer emotional distress to avoid demonstrating it or describing clear mental/behavioral symptoms to a physician. Rather, mental illness tends to be expressed to the doctor in somatic terms (e.g., aches, pains, fatigue), which are less stigmatizing. A result is confusion for the physician and difficulty in diagnosis. Here again, the EM affects care and outcome.

EMs are at the core of all illnesses. Along with their physical symptoms, patients bring their explanatory models to the physician's office or hospital. EMs are not left at home. By ignoring or minimizing the explanatory model, physicians or nurses tell patients that their beliefs about the problem that threatens their lives, lifestyles, or identities are irrelevant. Biomedicine's EM is more important than the patient's. This is a prescription for dissatisfaction.

Explanatory models, by the way, are a major reason why good explanations and smooth communication are essential in the clinical setting. Precisely because patients do present with their own ideas about cause and care, it is necessary to involve them in discussions of diagnosis, treatment, and prognosis. A brief, one-sided, professionally correct statement from the physician, nurse, technologist, or dietician about what is going on may be good for the professional ego but not for effective patient management.

Self-Treatment

With an explanatory model established, albeit only a preliminary one—EMs can evolve as symptoms change or worsen—the next step in the evolution of an illness is, typically, self-treatment. We all do this. It implies that we have made some preliminary diagnosis of our own—and we have. Our EMs direct us to the appropriate remedial action. The student with the possible kidney problem assumes he is just stiff from playing too hard (his EM) and takes some aspirin (the proper treatment, according to his EM). Maybe later he will try some Tylenol with codeine that a roommate or parent has in the medicine cabinet.

Very often, others are brought in for further help with diagnosis and prescribing. "Cousin Julia had symptoms similar to yours. It turned out to be such and such and she did so and so for it and it got better, so you take what Julia took." "Uncle Ben says your trouble in swallowing is probably a pulled nerve. You should gargle with salt water twice a day to neutralize it and it'll go away, so you try it." None of us rush to seek medical attention unless the symptoms are truly anxiety producing. Hot tea, chicken soup, chamomile, and laxatives—all are common responses to sickness. To this day, my sister is a firm believer that if you have diarrhea and nausea, then the best cure is plain rice and an active culture yogurt. But this means that she, like most of us, will not see a doctor until the situation lingers or gets worse. Thus, self-treatment has a significant effect on the disease that is ultimately presented to the physician or brought to the clinical setting for cure. In all cases, assume that the patient has self-treated before seeing the doctor or being admitted to the hospital.

Self-treatment and use of alternative medicine is not limited to ethnic groups. Americans of all ethnicities and social classes self-treat. Self-care items now constitute a significant part of Americans' overall healthcare expenses. Whether it is with herbs, prayers, magic, yogurt, teas, vitamins, or other over-the-counter health-food items, self-treatment by any patient can have an impact on the problem and its medical management. From the perspective of the biomedical professional, the result is the same. Self-treatment of any kind may delay "proper" medical treatment and can affect the course of the disease. When I worked at a large urban hospital, we often came across black diabetics who would self-treat before seeing a physician. Their EM for diabetes described it as being "sweet blood." Quite logically, this EM directed sufferers to treat the sweet blood by neutralizing the excess sweetness. Commonly used remedies included infusions of lemon juice or vinegar. Self-treatment here allowed the diabetes to worsen.

The reason self-treatment is so universal is that it typically works. The vast majority of sicknesses are self-limiting. No matter what you do for it, you eventually recover and give credit to the remedies you used at home or the therapists you visited. Even where the remedies fail, self-treatment strengthens the patient's identification with the illness and his or her responsibility in affecting it. If self-treatment is unsuccessful and the patient must ultimately seek biomedical help, then the patient has at least gained some owner-ship over the problem.

In most instances of sickness, the medical professional is the second choice and second line of recourse. Self-treatment almost always occurs first. A number of recent surveys indicate that more than 40 percent of Americans may use alternative therapies (e.g., herbals, chiropractors, acupuncturists, massage therapists, spiritual healers) for any given sickness (Cohen 2000; Eisenberg et al. 1998; Reed 1992, 68).

Ethnic group patients may have even more alternate professional resources. Some Puerto Ricans on the East Coast consult *espiritis-tas*. Miami Cubans may call upon a *santero*, Haitians a *hungan* or voodoo specialist. Some southern Blacks may contact a root doc-tor, Chicago Chinese an herbalist, Los Angeles or Denver Mexicans a *curandero*. Trust in formal, mainstream medical providers should not be taken for granted. Numerous reports suggest that Americans spend about as much money on alternate therapies as they do on formal medicine. Baby boomers are into herbals and supplements at an increasing rate.

The Sick Role

The illness continues to evolve. Symptoms have been identified (some accepted, others rejected as irrelevant), a tentative explana-tory model has been applied, and some form of self-treatment has been attempted. The sickness continues and begins to have an effect on the sufferer's activities. At this point, the individual may be ad-mitted to the sick role. The sick role defines the proper behavior for a sick person and officially identifies the sick person as a patient—at this point, a patient of the family, not yet of the physician or hospital. We all have these sick roles. They differ from family to family and ethnic group to ethnic group. Occupancy of the sick role confers certain rights and obligations. For example, if your child is crying and complaining of severe cramps at 7:30 in the morning, you may decide she does not have to go to school. She can stay in bed. You bring her food. You bring her a coloring book. You set up the portable TV on her dresser. She can cry and be irritable and far more demanding than usual and you tolerate it because it is appropriate. But for these privileges, she must be compliant (e.g., take the medicine you saved from last time, drink all of her tea), and she cannot skip out the door when her friends return from school, with a backward shout of "I'm feeling much better!"

On a more serious level, sick roles define the style of patienthood. Sick roles specify how demanding, complaining, or cooperative the patient should be, also how active or passive in attempting to get well, or how hopeful or fatalistic in attitude. EMs can affect sick-role behavior. The causes patients attribute illness to are " . . . important precisely because they reveal the meanings patients attach to those symptoms, disabilities, or diseases which they bring to the medical visit. And it is this meaning of illness that determines, in turn, the patient's illness behaviors, coping responses, and emotional reactions" (Stoeckle and Barsky 1981, 225). Thus, the sick role has a clear effect on your ability to manage that patient. Having some idea of the patient's sick role and orientation toward sickness can help you maximize the effectiveness of care provided.

Sick roles develop within families and ethnic groups. If you are sick, then you can and should exhibit these behaviors. The expressions of pain by the Italians, Jews, Irish, and Cubans mentioned previously all reflect the content of culturally prescribed and appropriate sick roles. Sick roles are rarely idiosyncratic expressions by patients. Rather, the demanding, complaining, or moaning, and the unrealistic cheerfulness, passivity, or denial are reflections of behaviors that are regularly rewarded by the patient's family and significant others. These behaviors were not invented just for the present hospital visit!

As with explanatory models, sick roles are brought to the hospital along with the medical problem. Of course, medical personnel have their own view of what constitutes a proper sick role for the hospitalized patient. The ideal patient should be compliant, forthcoming with information, collaborative, undemanding, un-complaining, and appreciative. Patients like this are "good" patients. They make medical management easier and more efficient. Patients who behave otherwise may be labeled as crocks or bad patients. Lorber's study (1975, 218) of a large New York City hospital demonstrated that nurses and physicians commonly labeled patients as good or problem. Good patients were cooperative, un-complaining, and stoical. Problem patients made trouble by complaining, being over-emotional, and dependent (see also Gordon 1983; Staley 1991). Labels can affect the behavior of those who do the labeling. Staff may take a bit more time in answering when a bad patient pushes the call button, or the interaction with a problem patient may be a bit cooler, with more formal professional demeanor and less empathy. Orders for psychological consults may be more likely.

Presenting the Illness to the Doctor

The decision to seek formal medical care is usually a complex one. Symptoms have been discussed with family or friends. Self-treatment is unsuccessful, and the patient has reached a threshold level of anxiety, discomfort, or inconvenience. For many, the decision to seek formal medical care is an economic one, where the anxiety and discomfort outweigh the financial implications of seeking formal care. For whatever reason, the medical consult or hospitalization has a certain imperative nature. The patient admits that the problem is beyond the control or realm of knowledge of self and significant others. Performance expectations of the physician or hospital are thus high.

Finally, the sick person stands before the physician. What does the patient tell the professional? Here, the patient sifts through everything that has already transpired. Perceived symptoms that seem appropriate to the situation are selected for presentation. Some symptoms may be dropped and others added. As mentioned earlier,

Kleinman (1980, 178–220) found that some Chinese mental patients focus on secondary physical complaints, not mentioning psychological problems or symptoms, mental illness being highly stigmatized in Chinese culture.

Physicians often ignore some of the patient's symptoms. The Western disease model of medicine classifies sicknesses into syndromes of co-occurring symptoms. A cold has symptoms of runny nose, sneezing, eye watering, and fatigue, among others, but not symptoms of eye twitching, nervousness, or numbness in the hand. Shingles may itch but not cause the patient to be "veak and dizzy." Physicians regularly ignore symptoms that do not seem relevant to medically familiar syndromes of disease. Or, once the physician has identified a key medical symptom, secondary symptoms—which can be of great importance to the patient—may be ignored.

For example, a young woman presents to the physician at an outpatient clinic. She complains of pains in both sides of her belly. Suspecting ovarian problems, the doctor's very first response to her symptom presentation is: "When did you have your last period, Miss Smith?" He then asks her about other urogenital problems. Here again, the initial presenting symptom (belly pain) is ignored, which tells the patient that her views and sensations are unimportant. In a sense, the doctor has co-opted her problem and turned it into *his*, not her, disease.

A fascinating ramification of this issue emerged from a study I did in Bogota, Colombia, on patterns of healthcare seeking by patients who use public medical outpatient clinics and patients who use *curanderos* (local folk healers). Both groups of patients were similar: largely rural migrants with low-paying blue collar jobs, a low level of formal education, and similar general health problems. When I interviewed both groups of patients, I elicited symptoms by asking, "What bothers you?" and prompting, "What else?" until no more symptoms were forthcoming. Patients at the folk healer's office listed an average of three or four symptoms. Patients at the outpatient clinic listed an average of six. Why the difference? Further interviews led me to conclude that patients added more symptoms at the clinic to ensure that at least one of the symptoms would be taken seriously and addressed by the physician. The *curandero* accepted all symptoms, rejecting none and addressing each. By producing more symptoms, the clinic patients were attempting to exert some personal control over the interaction and diagnosis. They anticipated that if they presented only a few symptoms, then the doctors might ignore these and create diseases of their own out of the patients' problems, thus co-opting the patients' sicknesses (Press 1969). Did the clinic patients actually have the additional symptoms? Probably, but all of us experience some discomforts in addition to the primary ones we present to our doctors.

Do patients lie to their physicians? Lots of times. Ask any doctor. Patients lie or hide things for many reasons. They may be afraid or ashamed to tell of the folk remedies they have already tried. In a fascinating study of physician/patient interaction in the rural south, Murphree and Barrow (1970) note that in every case they observed, the patient withheld information about use of old-time remedies they had taken prior to seeing the physician. More recently, Eisenberg et al. (1993, 244) finds similar behavior. He notes that "in more than seven of ten instances, users of unconventional therapy did not inform their medical doctor of their use of the therapy."

Patients may also hide symptoms. They may anticipate and fear the diagnosis or prognosis and avoid them by minimizing symptoms or severity. Misdirection is not necessarily a conscious ploy. A young medical resident related the following from the outpatient clinic:

> I had an old lady as a patient. She came in complaining of pain at the base of the spine, around the tailbone. I looked and tried everything I could, but wasn't able to diagnose anything. I thought she was goofy. Maybe a month later, she came back, this time complaining about pain just below the belly button. I poked and checked, but couldn't find a thing. Then, as part of a routine exam, I gave her a vaginal exam and found a serious infection. On a hunch, I turned her over and checked her anus. Sure enough, she had a significant problem there

as well. What I figured was that she viewed doctors as gods and was ashamed to trot out anal or vaginal problems for the "god" to see. So she moved the symptoms up out of the "naughty" areas to more neutral ground—the tailbone and the area just above the pubic hairline.

When patients omit information about self-treatment, or hide, shift, or reinterpret symptoms, it can affect the course of diagnosis and medical management—as well as the outcome. Thus, such omissions can affect satisfaction with care.

In addition to motives, the language used by patients to present their medical problem can have an effect on the interaction, diagnosis, and treatment. Physicians and nurses prefer articulate patients who can describe things clearly. "Doctor, I have this rather slowly growing pain in my left knee when I try to sleep on my right side, with my knees together. Also, I get a brief stabbing pain whenever I twist my knee to the left." Professionals much prefer this to "Doctor, my leg hurts a lot." Articulate patients with a good vocabulary may be treated with more respect and equality than an inarticulate patient who forces the physician to expend verbal effort in history taking. The physician's explanations and treatment options may be more forthcoming with the articulate patient than with the less verbal one.

A final and very important point about illness and the expression of symptoms to medical personnel: When someone—anyone—is sick, physical symptoms are only part of the problems that result. As suggested earlier, sickness can disrupt normal activities and roles. Plans are affected. Self-image is assaulted. This means that every sickness has social and emotional symptoms in addition to the somatic ones. These symptoms are also part of the illness. Patients at the folk healer's office often recite a list of symptoms such as, "Doctor, I have these belly pains, and a constant headache. I'm nervous all the time, and my business is not doing well." The healer accepts all of these as symptoms of a single syndrome. Would a typical physician? Patients in the doctor's office or hospital— whether in Bogota or Peoria—know that physicians and nurses will not take them seriously if they add the non-somatic symptoms they are suffering. Therefore, they fail to mention key factors that affect their well-being and cause anxiety in their daily lives. These disrupted aspects of daily lives are brought with the disease to the clinical setting, and they typically go unexpressed and unaddressed.

ROLES AND IDENTITIES

We are the sum total of our roles and identities. Without them, we are merely animals. These roles and identities—parent, child, spouse, coworker, neighbor, breadwinner, lover, friend, intellectual, delicate old person, jock, macho, sex pot, cool dude, fox, computer nerd—define who we are. All of these are simultaneously tucked down in our brains and activated as the context and situation requires. Interestingly, one of the few contexts where all or most of our roles and identities are consciously present is the hospital. This is because sickness threatens them all. It can make us unattractive. It weakens us and makes us less competent and appealing. When sick, we cannot work and provide or perform domestic tasks appropriately. We become a burden. We cannot meet our obligations to carpool the neighborhood kids so that our own kids get carpooled in turn. We miss the church meeting we were supposed to attend. Being sick and hospitalized takes us out of our normal contexts and makes meeting role obligations impossible.

Threats to roles and self-images accompany every patient and every disease to the hospital. These perceived threats and inconveniences are also part of the illness. The need for a clean room or warm food does not compare with guilt, anxiety, or embarrassment as issues of importance to patients.

On the Press Ganey inpatient survey, we ask patients to rate staff sensitivity to the problems and inconveniences that sickness and hospitalization can cause. Not surprisingly, this is invariably one of the top three issues most highly correlated with overall satisfaction with care across all hospitals. Treating the patient "like a real person" (a common yet ambiguous phrase) takes on clearer meaning in this context. The real person is threatened by having to be in your institution. Thus, effective empathy goes beyond concern for the physical comfort of the patient. Effective empathy must include sensitivity to the person who bears the disease and suffers the illness. When such sensitivity is lacking, the result can be distrust, patient perceptions of staff apathy, or perceived lack of a caring attitude on the part of staff. When such sensitivity is present, "it deepen(s) the therapeutic alliance that is at the heart of clinical care" (Levinson et al. 1997).

I remember observing an old lady in an ICU. She had tubes running out of every orifice, and she was very sick, but she was conscious. In their ministrations to her, staff repeatedly let her cover sheet slip off. They did not care, because they would be returning to her with frequency and keeping her naked was more efficient. Anyway, this was an ICU. Staying alive is the key issue—not dignity! The old lady would continuously and feebly reach down to attempt to pull the sheet back over her genital region. This very sick patient was concerned about her dignity and the staff were not. She had brought her identity and personality with her to the ICU. Of course, she was aware of and grateful for the heroic care she was receiving; however, the perceived assault to her dignity would likely modify her overall evaluation of this care.

Here's another example from my field notes while I was working with the consultation liaison psychiatry group:

June 23: We were called up to a medical floor by a young resident. His patient was an eighty-year-old black woman admitted through the ED with suspected congestive heart failure. His repeated attempts to convince her that she needed to have a blood gas draw had failed. "Mrs. Jones," he admonished, "we need to draw blood to see how much oxygen is getting to your system. It's important to know this. Now it won't hurt much."

No dice. "Nobody's sticking me!" she insisted. So he called for a psych consult. Up we come and, of course, the first thing she cries out when she sees our psychiatry department ID tags is the expected, "I'm not crazy!" Not surprisingly, she's now even more dissatisfied with care. While the young psych resident was talking with Mrs. Jones, I chatted with her two middle-aged daughters out in the hallway. Had momma ever been to a hospital before? No. Where were her five children delivered, then? At home. Her husband had died several years previously, and since that time she had become the matriarch of a large extended family. She was used to giving orders, not taking them. She assumed responsibility, not dependency. This hospital trip threatened her core identities.

I suggested that the resident try another approach. "Mrs. Jones," he said. "I'm only a resident here. I need to take a blood gas from you or I'll get in trouble. Please let me do it." This worked. Now she was back in charge. She agreed to the stick.

But not before she had been insulted by the psych consult. Psych consults are very often triggered by poor communication, not inherent psychiatric problems. In many instances, the psych consult is a cop-out, an indicator of failure by the medical staff to empathize with and understand the patient. To a significant extent, the barriers to patient compliance and collaboration with the staff lie in the roles and identities threatened by the medical problem, the hospitalization, and the treatment.

THE CLASH OF CULTURES

The evolution of an illness illustrates the complexity of the cultural baggage brought by the patient to the clinical encounter. Symptoms have been sensed and sorted through, some kept, and some dropped. Numerous interactions with significant others have confirmed suspicions, named the problem, and tentatively explained it and suggested courses of action. A sick role has been negotiated and legitimated within the family. Self-treatment has been attempted. The decision, typically negotiated with family, to seek formal medical care has been reached. Social, sexual, economic, and other roles have been affected, threatened, or impaired. All of this creates the illness that is brought to the physician or hospital along with any disease. Medical staff, however, are largely trained to recognize and deal with disease. A natural gap exists, and we are talking only about nonethnic, average American patients with English as their first language who were born and/or raised within the core American popular culture and medical system.

When significant ethnicity enters the picture, it becomes even more complex. Ethnic patients who maintain cultural elements from their country of origin bring additional cultural baggage. EMs become more distanced from common popular notions, as do concepts of healing and appropriate interaction with healthcare professionals. All cultures have their own traditional medical systems, regardless of whether Western medicine is officially present, and many elements of a different medical system may be maintained by some patients. Language barriers are often but the tip of the iceberg when it comes to establishing understanding, trust, and effective medical management for patients who bring a very different paradigm to the clinical encounter. Cultural as well as linguistic translation may be needed.

CONCLUSIONS

Although much of the preceding discussion is particularly relevant for the physician who must diagnose and devise appropriate treatment for patients, illness as a cultural construct accompanies every disease to the hospital and to some extent affects every patient's interaction with staff at all levels. We are not just talking about those staff who deal directly with diagnosing and treating the patient. Every delay, every aspect of body language or tone of voice that could be negatively interpreted, every miscue, every unexplained event or interruption—whether involving transport staff, volunteers, food service, housekeeping, nurses, physicians, or anyone else with whom the patient and family comes into contact—tells the patient that his or her problem or concerns are not being taken seriously.

The point of this discussion is to emphasize the complex nature of sickness. Food, amenities, cleanliness, and decor are important infrastructural elements. They certainly play a part in overall satisfaction. So, too, do technical competence and staff friendliness. But, to paraphrase George Orwell, all patient experiences in the hospital are equal, but some experiences are more equal than others. Patients bring significant cultural baggage—or illness—to the clinical encounter. Satisfaction with care depends to a large extent upon the manner in which staff deal with illness as opposed to the disease, which is clinically defined and technically managed. Not having been to medical or nursing school, patients can only judge clinical quality on the basis of actions and interactions that make sense to them. What makes sense is whatever addresses things that are important to them. Patients understand their illness quite well, even though they may not be able to articulate it in full.

Figure 4.1 ranks all items on the Press Ganey inpatient survey by their correlation with likelihood of recommending the hospital to others. Data were obtained from 2,178,000 patients rating care at 1,506 hospitals in 2004. A higher correlation coefficient means that the item is more highly linked to likelihood of recommending and has a stronger halo effect.

Food and amenities, while still significantly linked with satisfaction, are at the bottom of the list.

Note that the majority of items heading the list reflect illness and interaction rather than technical issues. Coordination of care, cheerfulness (ambience as well as staff interactions), service recovery, inclusion in decision making, information about what is being done, attention to dignity, sensitivity to the personal effect of sickness and hospitalization—these illness-relevant issues have most potential impact on patient satisfaction. The illness/disease distinction is a relevant concern for all who deal with patients, not just physicians.

Figure 4.1. Patient Satisfaction (Acute Care Inpatient) Correlated with Likelihood of Recommending Hospital

		Correlation with Likelihood to Recommend
1	How well staff worked together to care for you	0.79
2	Overall cheerfulness of the hospital	0.75
3	Response to concerns/complaints	0.69
4	Attention to special/personal needs	0.65
5	Sensitivity to inconvenience of health problems	0.65
6	Nurses kept you informed	0.64
7	Effort to include you in decisions	0.64
8	Nurses' attitude toward your requests	0.64
9	Skill of the nurses	0.63
10	Friendliness/courtesy of the nurses	0.62
11	Degree addressed emotional/spiritual needs	0.62

↓

40	How well things worked	0.40
41	Speed of admission	0.38
42	Temperature of the food	0.38
43	Noise level in and around room	0.37
44	Quality of the food	0.37
45	Room temperature	0.35

Note: n = 2,178,609 patients, 1,506 facilities; p < 0.001; Jan. 1–Dec. 31, 2004.
Source: Press Ganey Associates. 2004.

It must be stressed that to generate patient satisfaction, physicians, nurses, technologists, and others are not obliged to cede control of medical management to the patient by acquiescing to any EM or accommodating any behavior or special request for care. Explanations, serious listening, and empathy are key to patient satisfaction—not simply saying "yes" to any patient requests, ideas, and beliefs (Tuckett, Boutlon, and Williams 1985; Froehlich and Welch 1996).[1]

ACTION FOR SATISFACTION

1. Orient staff to the concept of patient culture. At the very least, all staff should receive a brief introduction to the concepts of sick roles and patient role/identity threats. These aspects of illness have a significant effect on the patient's behavior while in the hospital—that is, on medical management—and are typically expressed in the patient's interaction with a wide range of staff. Chaplains can be great training resources.

2. Respond to patients' symptoms. Listen. Address each symptom, in the order given. Explain why you are focusing on one rather than another of the patient's stated symptoms. This indicates you take the patient seriously and is a key to establishing trust. Many patients are eager to share their symptoms with others. After all, being sick and hospitalized is a major life event and verbalizing it is cathartic. All personnel should be coached to listen to patients if they want to talk.

3. Identify EMs. Attempt to elicit the patient's EM. Try to discern the implications of the EM. Discuss. Never disdain or belittle the patient's EM, but remember its importance to the patient. Explain the biomedical EM in clear language. Make sure the patient understands—a recitation of biomedical jargon will not help. Negotiate the EM, if possible, to obtain the patient's buy-in to the diagnosis and proposed treatment. Remember that this is not medical school and the patient is not a medical student. It is not really important if the negotiated EM is not quite standard medicine, as long as the patient begins to feel at ease with the management program that is appropriate. If the patient does not buy into your EM, then dissatisfaction—and noncompliance—are likely to result.

   Responding to all symptoms and eliciting the patient's EM is important. When the physician co-opts the patient's problem by imposing the biomedical symptomology and EM, the disease is then owned by the physician. This is an important concept, because it suggests that if there is any problem (e.g., error, complication, comorbidity, poor outcome), then the physician or hospital is at fault because responsibility for the disease as well as its cure has been taken from the patient.

4. Understand self-treatment. Elicit what the patient has done for the problem. Everyone self-treats. Get an idea of what the patient thought would work. Do not put down their self-treatment, which might easily reflect long-held family or cultural traditions that the patient respects. Indicate that the self-treatment reflects a logical response to the patient's EM—thus, the patient does not feel belittled and trust can be established in the biomedical EM and in the appropriate treatment. Approving of harmless self-treatments the patient appears to favor (and even recommending them when the patient returns home) may encourage trust and compliance with the biomedical regimen.

5. Use patients' sick roles to facilitate medical management. Unless the patient is downright disruptive, work with their behaviors insofar as possible. Remember that the sick-role behaviors expressed are likely viewed as appropriate and are rewarded by the patient's family and significant others. These behaviors are called *roles* for a reason. They are learned and habitual. They provide the patient with a familiar script for expressing anxieties, fears, and needs in the unfamiliar, threatening clinical context. Retraining, or subtly punishing the patient for inappropriate behavior, is not the staff's responsibility. Staff must discuss ways in which patient behaviors can be accommodated without judging them to be examples of "acting out," which is an official negative term describing inappropriate behavior. By labeling patients as acting out, we remove their credibility.

6. Acknowledge roles and identities. Staff must be sensitized to the need to elicit patient concerns not only about the course of treatment, but also about the effect of the disease and hospitalization on their lives and perceptions of self. All hospital staff empathize with patients; however, to have an

effect, this empathy must be perceived by the patient. Hospital staff can easily shift into a clinical mentality. This mode of thinking includes such concepts as those included in the following example:

Good patients should leave their personal problems at home. They should not bother us by pushing the call button too frequently. They should be compliant, undemanding, trusting, quiet, and grateful. They should not be concerned with trivia such as personal dignity. After all, they are sick and this is a hospital.

This mentality has been responsible all these years for the embarrassing short gowns (an assault to personal dignity), the use of first names rather than "Mr." or "Ms.," the labeling of patients as good or bad, the turfing of problem patients to psychiatry or social work practitioners, and so forth.

7. Be aware of cultural diversity (ethnicity) as a complicating factor. Staff must have some familiarity with the medical beliefs and expectations of ethnic groups that have a significant representation among your patients. If every interaction between patient and provider is a form of cultural transaction, then ethnicity obviously complicates it further. See the next chapter for a more complete discussion of diversity.

NOTE

1. Physicians may find it quite useful to review Platt's discussions (1992; 1995) of good and bad doctor/patient communication. His verbatim examples of history-taking illustrate many of the principles discussed in this chapter and the potential therapeutic consequences of (not) understanding where the patient's coming from.

REFERENCES

Cohen, J. J. 2000. "Reckoning with Alternative Medicine." *Academic Medicine* 75 (6): 571.

Cohen, L. M. 1979. *Culture, Disease and Stress Among Latino Immigrants*. RIIES Special Study. Washington, DC: Research Institute on Immigration and Ethnic Studies, Smithsonian Institution.

Eisenberg, D. M., R. B. Davis, S. L. Ettner, S. Appel, S. Wilkey, M. Van Rompay, and R. C. Kessler. 1998. "Trends in Alternative Medicine Use in the United States, 1990–1997: Results of a Follow-up National Survey." *JAMA* 280 (18): 1569–75.

Eisenberg, D. M., R. C. Kessler, C. Foster, F. E. Norlock, D. R. Calkins, and T. L. Delbanco. 1993. "Unconventional Medicine in the United States: Prevalence, Costs, and Patterns of Use." *New England Journal of Medicine* 328 (4): 246–52.

Eisenberg, L. 1977. "Diseases and Illness: Distinctions Between Professional and Popular Ideas of Sickness." *Culture, Medicine and Psychiatry* 1 (1): 9–23.

Froehlich, G. W., and H. G. Welch. 1996. "'Meeting Walk-in Patients' Expectations for Testing: Effects on Satisfaction." *Journal of General Internal Medicine* 11 (8): 470–74.

Gordon, D. 1983. "Hospital Slang for Patients: Cracks, Gomers, Gorks, and Others." *Language in Society* 12 (2): 173–85.

Kleinman, A. 1987. "Explanatory Models in Health-Care Relationships: A Conceptual Frame for Research on Family-Based Health-Care Activities in Relation to Folk and Professional Forms of Clinical Care." MIT Press Series on the Humanistic and Social Dimensions of Medicine, no. 5. In *Encounters Between Patients and Doctors: An Anthology*, edited by J. D. Stoeckle, 273–83. Cambridge, MA: MIT Press.

Kleinman, A. 1980. *Patients and Healers in the Context of Culture*. Berkeley, CA: University of California Press.

Kleinman, A., L. Eisenberg, and B. Good. 1978. "Culture, Illness, and Care: Clinical Lessons from Anthropologic and Cross-Cultural Research." *Annals of Internal Medicine* 88 (2): 251–58.

Lambert, W., E. Libman, and E. Poser. 1960. "The Effect of Increased Salience of a Membership Group on Pain Tolerance." *Journal of Personality* 38: 350–57.

Lorber, J. 1975. "Good Patients and Problem Patients: Conformity and Deviance in a General Hospital." *Journal of Health and Social Behavior* 16 (2): 213–25.

Levinson, W., D. Roter, J. Mullooly, V. Dull, and R. Frankel. 1997. "Physician-Patient Communication: The Relationship with Malpractice Claims among Primary Care Physicians and Surgeons." *JAMA* 277 (7): 553–59.

Murphree, A. H., and M. V. Barrow. 1970. "Physician Dependence, Self-Treatment Practices, and Folk Remedies in a Rural Area." *Southern Medical Journal* 63 (4): 403–08.

Platt, F. W. 1995. *Conversation Repair: Case Studies in Doctor-Patient Communication*. Boston: Little, Brown.

Platt, F. W. 1992. *Conversation Failure: Case Studies in Doctor-Patient Communication*. Tacoma, WA: Life-Sciences Press.

Press, I. 1969. "Urban Illness: Physicians, Curers, and Dual Use in Bogota." *Journal of Health and Social Behavior* 10 (3): 209–17.

Reed, J. C. 1992. "Alternative Systems of Medical Practice." In *Alternative Medicine: Expanding Medical Horizons*. Report to the National Institutes of Health on Alternative Medical Systems and Practice in the United States. Chantilly, VA: Workshop on Alternative Medicine.

Staley, J. C. 1991. "Physicians and the Difficult Patient." *Social Work* 36 (1): 74–79.

Stoeckle, J., and A. Barsky. 1981. "Attributions: Uses of Social Science Knowledge in the 'Doctoring' of Primary Care." In *The Relevance of Social Science for Medicine*, edited by L. Eisenberg and A. Kleinman, 223–40. Dudrecht, Holland: D. Reidel.

Tuckett, D., C. O. Boutlon, and A. Williams. 1985. *Meetings Between Experts: An Approach to Sharing Ideas in Medical Consultations*. London: Tavistock.

Zborowski, M. 1952. "Cultural Components in Responses to Pain." *Journal of Social Issues* 8 (4): 16–30.

Zola, I. K. 1966. "Culture and Symptoms: An Analysis of Patients' Presenting Complaints." *American Sociological Review* 31 (5): 615–30.

CHAPTER 5

Dealing with Cultural Diversity

THE CASE FOR CULTURAL COMPETENCE IN HEALTHCARE

Thus far, we have been discussing patient culture as though it were a solitary, homogeneous entity confronting the equally homogeneous entity of the hospital culture. In truth, patients can vary dramatically in their medical beliefs and practices. Staff, too, exhibit considerable variation in cultural background and familiarity with American healthcare professional roles.

Culture refers to a cohesive body of learned behaviors, taught from one generation to the next. One's culture constitutes one's rationale and rules for living. Culture makes experiences meaningful. Cultures are not simply a hodgepodge of disparate habits. They are full-blown, patterned systems of regulations for interpreting and responding to events. This means that (1) they are immensely important to their bearers; (2) they engender resentment if challenged; and (3) they are hard to change.

Cultural clashes occur in a variety of contexts. Nowhere, however, are the stakes as high as in healthcare.

During the few hours or days the patient is in your care, you will not be able to change his or her habits and values. The trick is to accommodate the patient's culture to enhance patient satisfaction and maximize the effectiveness of your medical intervention.

To question someone's culture is to threaten it—and him or her. As indicated earlier, all cultures reflect the knowledge that sickness can mean disability, disfigurement, familial and social disruption, psychological stress, economic hardship, or death. All cultures contain medical systems that explain sickness and offer rules and roles for coping with it. Thus, the variant beliefs, practices, and expectations of care contained by these systems lie at the very core of the patients' and their families' world views. If these beliefs and expectations are not addressed or accommodated by hospital staff, then the result can be distrust, reticence, and noncompliance.

It takes two parties to create a cultural gap. In Chapter 3, we noted that the hospital itself constitutes a culture that gives meaning to the work and identity of its staff. Both staff and patients approach the clinical encounter with deeply held ideas about what is best for the patient. Patients who feel that their particular needs—medical or otherwise—are not being met may actively attempt to thwart what staff view as essential care. Or patients may appear to passively accept this care, while internally denying its legitimacy and withholding questions, doubts, and even essential information from the caregivers.

It is not just treatment in the hospital that is at stake. Many patients return home while still requiring daily medications, therapy, and exercises to complete their recuperation. Thus, outcome itself, or at least speed of recovery, can be affected. Patients dissatisfied by a lack of culturally sensitive medical management while in the hospital are more likely to be noncompliant once home. As Pachter (1994, 690) notes

> It can be expected that appropriate use of health services, compliance with therapeutic interventions and improved health outcomes

have a higher likelihood of being realized when the healthcare provider and the patient acknowledge and respect each other's beliefs about illness, even though these beliefs may not be wholly concurrent.

Experienced healthcare providers are well aware that beliefs and practices can vary all over the map. Some appear exotic, some outright bizarre to us. Many seem useless and scientifically invalid. Many patients' requests or practices appear to be social, with no relationship to the issue (sickness) at hand. This is because patients bring their *whole* culture to the hospital—not merely their medical systems. They arrive with their languages, dietary preferences, dignity and privacy expectations, rules for hospitality, interaction with strangers or authority figures, and a host of other habits and needs. Easily viewed as noise by harried staff, these phenomena constitute the essential context of life for patients.

Betancourt, Green, and Carrillo (2002) suggest that "Cultural competence in healthcare describes the ability of systems to provide care to patients with diverse values, beliefs and behaviors, *including tailoring delivery to meet patients' social, cultural and linguistic needs*"(emphasis added). This definition recognizes that staff must meet more than the linguistic or somatic/medical needs of patients. If sociocultural and emotional (as well as medical) needs go unmet because a cultural gap between patient and staff is not adequately addressed, then the result may be reduced medical competence as well.

All of this reflects the fact that a roster of interpreters does not in itself constitute a diversity program.

Cultural differences can go far beyond language. Some religious groups (e.g., orthodox Jews, Jehovah's Witnesses, Seventh Day Adventists) typically have no language issues but bring significantly diverse beliefs to the hospital. Scheduling conferences or procedures between sundown on Friday through sundown on Saturday can create major difficulties for Orthodox Jews. They might not be able to travel by car and could not take elevators to upper hospital floors. But they speak English.

WHO IS CULTURALLY DIVERSE?

There is no question that our country is becoming more culturally heterogeneous. There has been constant migration, and there are plenty of folks for whom English is a second language and American a second culture. The famous melting pot often takes two or three generations to dissolve foreign backgrounds into the general culture.

We tend to equate cultural diversity with ethnicity. It is true that the most exotic variant health beliefs and practices are brought to the hospital by patients from other countries. Many migrants come from countries and regions where modern clinical medicine is scarce or absent and where folk practitioners and non-Western medical systems are the rule. Preventive medicine is unfamiliar. One goes to healers only when one is sick. Explanatory models may differ dramatically from Western clinical causal and treatment concepts. Self-treatment is common. Physicians and hospitals are a last resort, because they are unfamiliar and assumed to be expensive.

If only diversity were this simple!

Being born in (or having parents born in) another country does not automatically equate to language or behavioral variance. We probably all know Mexicans, Italians, Japanese, or Koreans who do not speak a word of their mother tongues. The only thing ethnic about them is their name—and sometimes, not even that. At the same time, even if your patient speaks no English, you cannot assume he or she is unsophisticated in the basics of Western medicine or behavioral customs.

Nationality-based ethnicity, of course, is not the only source of variant beliefs and behaviors. Even being 100 percent American does not guarantee that a patient is familiar with the language and concepts of medicine. Each U.S. region nurtures subcultures that differ from the standard American to varying degrees. Rural dwellers from certain states may exhibit significant stoicism and lack of cooperation during medical care, as well as exhibiting some variant medical beliefs.

An important source of diversity often overlooked by clinical staff is socio-economic status. If patients look and sound like "real" Americans, then it is easy to assume that they share basic health concepts and language with providers. Most physicians, nurses, and technologists are middle class or higher. Street culture may be as foreign to them as any exotic nationality. Moreover, for many staff members, the "culture of poverty" (e.g., Lewis 1959) exhibited by some patients is as exotic as any nationality-based behavioral system. People living with chronic poverty may exhibit distrust of authority, hopelessness, and a present-time orientation that interferes with their ability to plan for the future. Add vocabulary and educational insufficiencies to this, and you may have a recipe for poor information exchange and lack of active cooperation and compliance with clinical regimens—both during treatment and after discharge.

Cultural diversity thus has a number of causes as well as a number of behavioral manifestations. Whether based on nationality, region, youth culture, street culture, or poverty, variant beliefs and lifestyles can affect diagnosis, medical management, patient comfort, and outcome.

RESPONDING TO DIVERSITY

The more at ease the patient—and family—the more you have working for you. As noted in the first chapter, patients who are more satisfied with their care are more likely to be compliant, cooperative, and positively responsive to your medical management. Patient satisfaction concerning care is also affected by their take on your response to their idiosyncratic requests for not-in-the-nursing-textbook care.

This non-textbook care includes any alternative medical interventions or elements of care felt by patients or families to be appropriate. These interventions can range from simple dietary requests to the outright bizarre.

Most requests by patients and families will likely be nonmedical or will not interfere with necessary treatment and care. Note the word "necessary"; it describes interventions that are essential to ameliorating or healing the patient's sickness. In this sense, issues relating to food preferences, accommodations, modesty, and family behavior are not "necessary."

We must rethink the definition of nondisruptive. It is easy to label almost any unorthodox request by the patient or family as disruptive insofar as it requires staff time (e.g., "to keep an eye on what they're doing") or contradicts clinical rituals relating to hygiene, housekeeping, and expectations of appropriate behavior by visitors.

Note that the phrase "clinical rituals" was used here. *Ritual* implies automatic, customary behavior whose value is taken for granted. Ritual is sacred in the sense that "this is the way we've always done it," implying that the behavior is naturally appropriate. Rituals typically originate as useful behaviors. Over time, the initial functions may become obsolete, yet the behaviors continue as rituals. Rituals in the clinical setting were often created in the first place to make care more efficient and convenient for the caregiver— not necessarily better for the patient. Any routine aspect of care that can inconvenience or dissatisfy patients should be examined for its *present* functional contribution to patient care as opposed to staff convenience. There are so many care protocols (rituals) that are at least partially based on convenience versus medical necessity that some amount of compromise or negotiation is usually possible:

> An example: An elderly Middle Eastern woman dies in the hospital. Her family crowds into her room and begins to wail and cry around the body, creating considerable stress on the unit. In Middle Eastern culture, such outpourings and gathering around the corpse are an important and ritualized part of mourning. You can either demand silence and/or usher all or most of the family out (this would be hospital ritual) or you can move the body to a private area to

accommodate the family's need for time and space to mourn loudly. Unless the patient died of something extremely contagious, this response contradicts no clinically essential protocol and generates much good will.

Another example: Some Mexicans believe that a coin should be taped to the umbilicus of a newborn baby to prevent a bulging bellybutton. Nurses may object to this, being concerned about the possibility of infection. However, if a coin is sterilized in alcohol first, then it will not compromise the baby's health and will make the parents feel a lot better about the hospital's understanding.

There is little that most alternative modes of care can do to actually harm the patient while he or she is in the hospital. Unless the patient requires a very sterile environment (most patients do not and most hospital rooms are not), almost anything that is not outright disruptive will not affect your medical management. Visitors are probably less likely than staff to transmit dangerous infections through touching and bringing outside items into contact with the patient. Of course, no interventions, foods, or folk remedies should be allowed without a physician's or nurse's approval!

You do not have to compromise or negotiate basic biomedical care. But if there are viable treatment alternatives compatible with the patient's particular beliefs, then negotiation is possible. Earlier, we discussed the importance of the EMs that patients bring to the clinical setting. These EMs are taken very seriously. A common Mexican explanatory model defines diarrhea as a cold disease, best treated with a hot remedy. Penicillin is defined as cold, and logically would thus exacerbate rather than cure the diarrhea. However, if mixed with chocolate (viewed as hot), then the penicillin is warmed and thus made effective. Here (assuming oral penicillin will be an effective medical treatment), negotiation can result in reduced anxiety, enhanced trust, and greater satisfaction.

Some requests will be difficult, if not impossible, to accommodate. For example, if the patient or family indicates that the bed should be moved because its orientation with respect to the window or door is unlucky, then there is probably little you can do. However, there may be other, minor furniture changes that could neutralize the unlucky positioning of the bed. If you cannot accommodate the patient's request, then ask whether there is something else that can be done to make the situation better. A bit of redecorating will probably not interfere with essential protocols of clinical care.

Negotiation does not undermine your authority or professional identity. Rather, it enhances these by marking you as caring, sensitive and unprejudiced.

IDENTIFYING VARIANT PATIENT NEEDS

The complex nature of diversity itself creates difficulties for hospital staff who wish to accommodate the special cultural needs of patients. How do you determine which patients need accommodating? Asking a Chinese patient, regardless of her facility with English, whether she would like chopsticks with dinner could be insulting, depending upon her degree of acculturation. At the same time, she may indeed desire chopsticks but may be too intimidated or embarrassed to directly ask for them.

A culturally competent program must have a means of identifying patients with special cultural needs and determining whether language, beliefs, or family practices require special mediation.

It can be useful to present a checklist of needs to *all* patients or their families as soon as possible after admission. The advantage of such a list is that it has a chance of eliciting special culture-based needs without appearing to stereotype the patient by race, social class, or nationality. Moreover, even if the patient is reticent about responding, the very act of posing such questions demonstrates the hospital's interest in and openness to accommodating special needs. An initial cultural assessment can save much nursing time. Knowing what the patient will or will not eat, drink (e.g., ice in the water glass), or do can prevent duplicated trips and interventions and can enhance cooperation.

This kind of checklist can also reveal whether technical or personal aspects of care need to be negotiated, whether staff should bring in an ethnic ombudsman, or consult the ethnicity library— your collection of books and articles on various ethnic groups' medical beliefs and practices. Even if your patient clearly requires an interpreter, poor English facility does not equate to possession of exotic medical beliefs and care needs. At the same time, any patient (not just ethnics) may have idiosyncratic personal care needs or medical beliefs that, if unaddressed, can lead to increased anxiety and dissatisfaction. Thus, a general checklist can be useful for all patients. It should be translated into all major languages of your patient constituency. Interpreters working with patients on this checklist should be able to pick up hints about specific needs and probe more deeply into these issues.

The following list of enquiries is not complete and is meant to be suggestive only. Examples in parenthesis are for illustrative purposes, to indicate the types of needs that might be discovered.

Meals
1. Is there anything you need to do before you eat? (prayers, hand or mouth washing)
2. Do you require any special utensils for eating?
3 Are there any foods you do not want to eat? (pork, meat, eggs, dairy with meat dishes, cold foods or liquids)
4. Are there any foods you want with each meal? (rice, hot sauce, tea)
5. Is there anything you need to do after you eat? (prayers, hand or mouth washing)

Room
1. Would you like one of these wall hangings* in your room?
2. Is there something else you would like to have in your room?
3. Is there something we should change or remove in the room?

Medical care

1. Is there something we should not do (to you)? (bathing, blood draws or transfusions)
2. Is there any medicine we should not give you? ("cold" substances, alcohol-based)
3. Is there something we should definitely do?
4. Is there anything your family can do for you here to help you get better? (feeding, washing, massages, amulets, prayers, presence during examinations, bringing in a healer)
5. Does it matter whether a male or female nurse or doctor takes care of you?
6. Is there any special type of practitioner you think should be brought in to help you? (religious practitioner, folk healer)

Discharge

1. Is there anything special you need to do before leaving?
2. [To family]: Are you able to perform the kinds of care that the patient requires at home? (bathing, wound dressing changes, medications at specified times. Note: depending upon the ethnic group, fathers or sons may be unwilling or culturally unable to assist a daughter or mother with hygienic care or anything relating to her breasts, genitals or anus.)

*An aside on wall hangings: Decor is important. It can affect mood and stress level. Offer *all* patients a choice of one piece of art for their room. I am talking about inexpensive prints, although original art could also be offered—ask local artists to donate or lend pieces of their work to the hospital. Present a printed menu page with photos of the pictures, or have the patient view these on the room TV. The prints or art works should represent a variety of meaningful (not abstract) scenes—the sea, desert, forest, mountains, flowers, cornfields, or exotic settings. Such images evoke more meaningful and calming emotional responses than do abstract works. It is essential to also include prints of prayer in appropriate languages and religious imagery from various major religions, including Judaism, Islam, Christianity, Buddhism, and Hinduism. Many patients will feel more at ease with a religious image or text on the wall. All patients will appreciate the opportunity to select a familiar or soothing scene or landscape. By representing both secular and sacred images among the art offerings, you avoid stereotyping while offering patients an important therapeutic contextual element.

CREATING A PROGRAM

Let's face it—you are not going to make cultural anthropologists out of your staff. There is no way they can memorize all the variant beliefs and practices of the many different patient groups you serve. At the same time, staff must be made aware of and familiar with—and at ease with—the fact that there may be great diversity in beliefs and practices relating to sickness and healing among the different patient constituencies they serve. Some familiarity with specific ethnic or religious group beliefs or practices relating to certain common conditions or procedures (e.g., heart attack, childbirth, diabetes) should be fostered among staff who regularly deal with these issues.

For example, if you have a large Mexican patient constituency, then obstetric nurses should be aware of a common belief that postpartum women should avoid baths and drafts because the uterus is open and susceptible to bad winds, or *vientos*, that can get up into the mother and cause harm. Many Asian groups believe that new mothers should stay out of drafts and avoid cold liquids. Many groups place amulets near or on the baby for good luck.

Regular in-service presentations on the healthcare beliefs and needs of specific ethnic or social groups will reinforce the importance of cultural competence, while increasing sensitivity to patient differences. Nurses from various ethnic groups could be asked to discuss the special needs of patients who share their cultural background. Many medical anthropologists specialize in the health beliefs and practices of different cultures; contact your local university to identify potential speakers.

Bring in several laypeople of each ethnic group you serve to act as voluntary consultants. A good source would be a religious institution (e.g., church, mosque, temple, synagogue). Show them patient rooms and equipment. Describe a typical patient's care trajectory, including donning the hospital gown and bed pan use. Describe procedures. If you can get some patients to agree to being observed during certain procedures (e.g., giving meds, taking vitals, IV insertions, meal delivery), then so much the better. Debrief these volunteer consultants, asking them to identify any experience that might be problematic for patients of their ethnic group. Also ask for their suggestions on how to modify patient experiences. Present the information at in-services for staff. Create booklets for your cultural reference library.

This library should contain observations, books, articles, and video support materials on cultural diversity. There are many written sources available. Because of their depth and specificity, most materials are more useful as background resources than as guides for day-to-day patient care management. Again, do not expect staff to memorize the detailed medical beliefs of multiple ethnic groups. A number of books and articles describe, in great detail, the health beliefs and practices of specific population groups (e.g., African Americans, Mexicans, Puerto Ricans, Haitians, Navajos, Chinese, Laotians). A medical anthropologist at your local university could provide a specialized list of recommended articles and books that would not ordinarily show up in professional healthcare bibliographies.

The University of Washington Medical Center has developed a series of short (one or two pages) tip sheets for easy reviewing by staff when dealing with any of 11 different types of patients. These Culture Clues™ are available online for anyone to use with proper attribution.

Programs for Specific Patient Constituencies

There should be a plan in place to handle special patient needs—both medical and nonmedical. Most hospitals already have frozen kosher meals available for orthodox Jewish patients, or vegetarian offerings for Hindus. Anticipating symbolically important needs of different groups can have a strong influence on their satisfaction with care. For example, identifying the eastern wall of their rooms exhibits your sensitivity to accommodating the prayer needs of Muslim patients.

If one of your larger patient constituencies experiences a particular heath issue, then it is essential to develop programs to address them.

Several years ago, Sinai-Grace Hospital in Detroit, Michigan, began development of a bloodless treatment program for the treatment of an increasing number of Jehovah's Witness patients. The decision was made partly as a response to the number of Witnesses who used the hospital and partly as a strategic marketing decision to become the hospital of choice for members of this religious group, a significant number of whom live in the Detroit area.

Program developers first met with leaders of the religious group to learn more about their treatment needs. The hospital identified both nurses and physicians who were willing to accommodate Witness treatment beliefs in various medical specialties (e.g., oncology, surgery, labor and delivery). A separate consent form was developed for patients declining transfusions or use of blood products. Arguments were prepared for treatment negotiation (e.g., justification of why platelets and plasma might be viable alternatives to real blood). It was noted that, like many groups, Jehovah's Witnesses were not homogeneous, some being less conservative than others.

The Hospital for Special Surgery, in New York City, has developed culturally sensitive programs that target Hispanics and Chinese suffering from lupus. Brochures in Spanish and Chinese tell patients about the disease and stress that it is not the patient's fault, thus addressing common Chinese EMs about personal causality.

As both Hispanics and Chinese tend to place importance on self-treatment with herbals, the brochures warn that some alternative treatments can be harmful. For example, the Chinese brochure is quite specific in its recognition that patients may also be using traditional medicine.

> Many Chinese patients use traditional Chinese medicine as part of their treatment. Acupuncture and Tai Chi have been known to reduce joint pain and lower stress. However, you should not rely on these treatments alone. Traditional Chinese medical doctors will prescribe herbal medicines, but we don't know enough about how they might help or harm the body. Therefore, it is important to tell your doctor about all of the treatments you are using, both Western and Chinese medicine.

Ethnic Ombudsmen

Beyond brochures, however, understanding and compliance can be significantly enhanced if counseling can be provided by fellow ethnics who were or who are presently being treated for the same medical problem.

Such an ombudsman is familiar with specific clinical processes and procedures. He or she can explain illnesses, treatments, and hospital protocols to patients. An ideal ombudsman, of course, is a nurse of the patient's own ethnic group. However, it would be most useful for the hospital to have a cadre of volunteer former patients to counsel fellow ethnic patients about diseases or procedures they themselves have experienced.

The Hospital for Special Surgery, in New York City, has created several unusual programs that use Hispanic, Chinese, and African American lupus sufferers to counsel patients. Both the Hispanic "Charla de Lupus" and the Chinese "LANtern" (Lupus Asian Network) programs train bilingual lupus sufferers to serve as peer health educators. These volunteers answer questions about the disease and counsel patients about treatment modes and lifestyle accommodations. As fellow ethnics, they know many of the traditional beliefs that can impede understanding of the nature and treatment of the disease. An important aspect of this program is the fact that these ombudsmen are nonprofessionals. They avoid being stigmatized as authorities, such as doctors or nurses, thus encouraging questions, discussion, and compliance.

Interpreters

Sometimes, you simply have to use whoever is available. If you have a choice, however, then be careful about the interpreter's gender and age. Obviously, you will want to match gender with the patient if at all possible. But age is also an issue. Translators that appear too young may be counterproductive. Educated college students may be bilingual in English and their ethnic group's language, but their youth can easily discourage adults from discussing personal issues. Many adults of almost any ethnic group will be very hesitant to talk about personal matters with people of an obviously younger generation. If a patient brings in a grandchild to translate for him or her—a common situation, in that grandchildren are likely born and educated in the United States—then do not count on getting the patient's full story. As a general rule, do not use family members to translate for the patient if a qualified interpreter is available.

Apart from official interpreters, you should keep a roster of individuals in your organization who can speak different languages. Note their departments, work hours, and pager or phone numbers. They can be called upon in emergent situations to help with translation. This is preferable to using family members, because these staff are not emotionally involved and likely are more familiar with medical terms and processes and can explain them with greater clarity.

The interpreter, of course, is a person as well as a resource. This person has an impact on the patient. Gender, age, appearance, and accent can affect the level of candor and accuracy of history taking and explanations. Many languages also have regional or social class variants that can identify the speaker as an outsider. For example, an obvious New York accent can be unpleasant to a deep southerner, or a cockney accent grating to an upper-middle-class Londoner. Accent differences can potentially make any patient ill at ease, even with a translator of his or her own nationality. The result can be an incomplete exchange of information.

Although it is more likely that upper income or more highly educated ethnic patients speak some English and are more familiar with modern medical concepts and vocabulary, if you have a choice, try to recruit translators whose accents and vocabulary are more general to better communicate with the rest of your patient population.

STAFF DIVERSITY

A culturally diverse staff can have an impact on care as well as on both patient and employee satisfaction. According to *Hospitals and Health Networks* (Mills-Senn 2005, 30), the number of foreign-born nurses in U.S. hospitals jumped from 9 percent in the mid 1990s to 12 percent of the workforce today. The number continues to grow as a nursing shortage continues. Responding to this shortage, in May of 2005, Congress authorized the issuance of additional visas for recruitment of nurses from the Philippines, India, China, and other countries that have exceeded their visa quotas.

Politically correct or not, it is a fact that the nationality, race, and ethnicity of nurses, physicians, and technologists can affect interaction with patients. People tend to trust professionals who look and talk like them. Nurses who cannot speak or understand vernacular English with ease may cause gaps or errors in the exchange of information with patients. Many patients—especially those from other countries—have a hard enough time communicating in English without having to deal with someone who speaks English with a marked accent and "awkward" vocabulary. Moreover, elderly patients with hearing problems can have difficulty understanding the questions and instructions of nurses and physicians with strong accents.

Patients may generally feel more at ease with staff who share their cultural identity. But this is human nature, so the same goes for staff, as well. Nurse behaviors that are quite normal in other countries may be viewed as strange or unprofessional by American-trained nurses. Moreover, racial, national, and ethnic stereotypes can have an impact on the manner and effectiveness of staff interaction with one another.

Let's face it: Prejudice exists among healthcare professionals as well as the general public. Americans are as chauvinistic as any other people in the world and often view professional training in modestly industrialized nations as second-rate. Both patients and staff may distrust the competence of nurses with different physical features, marked accents, and English deficiencies.

Behavioral and personality characteristics of foreign staff can stimulate resentment and distrust. Some foreign-born nurses view physicians, supervisors, and administrators as authority figures whom it is inappropriate to approach with questions or suggestions. Recent migrants may feel reluctant about demonstrating their ignorance by asking questions. To colleagues, however, this may appear to be arrogance or indifference. In some cultures, avoidance of eye contact is a sign of politeness and deference—not inattention or disrespect. Various cultures, particularly many Asian cultures, stress that women should be respectful of age and authority and should avoid confrontation and shaming others. This can result in poor leadership skills (by American standards) as well as perceptions (by colleagues) of professional inadequacy. In short, behavioral and personality traits generated in other cultures can create failures or delays in communication and trust when exhibited in a U.S. hospital setting.

Let's agree that your patients deserve the best of care. Ideally, political correctness should be secondary to clinical and interpersonal effectiveness. We must assume that the nurses you hire are clinically competent and have met appropriate standards of knowledge, or they would not be accredited at your hospital in the first place. However, a clinically competent nurse who is nonetheless unfamiliar with American sex roles, professional roles, and the hospital organization and who speaks English with a significant accent and variant vocabulary may be more likely to generate poor communication (with colleagues as well as patients), delays, and even errors.

You will want to address staff diversity in a number of ways, such as the following.

1. Prepare a standard interview protocol, both verbal and written, to ascertain a foreign applicant's proficiency with English (including common hospital slang), clarity of pronunciation, and familiarity with the U.S. hospital organization. As noted, the workloads, job performance standards, and lines of authority experienced by nurses in their home countries may differ significantly from common U.S. expectations. Indeed, a recent report indicates that many foreign-born nurses have never even worked in a hospital before (Mills-Senn 2005, 31).

2. Establish a program for mentoring and acculturating foreign-born staff. In-service workshops should be presented on topics such as nurse/physician interaction, nurse/supervisor interaction, collegiality, responding to errors, and asking for help. Assign each new foreign-born nurse to a mentor, a U.S.-born or experienced fellow nurse (ideally of the same nationality) to give advice, to explain work roles and departmental politics, and to act as a go-between with physicians and even supervisors during the early months on the job.

3. Establish a program for your American-born nurses that discusses relevant cultural traditions of countries that supply significant numbers of your foreign-born staff. Here, a foreign nurse with many years of U.S. hospital experience could be an ideal presenter. Each issue of your inhouse employee newsletter should spotlight your new foreign-born and trained nurses, describing their backgrounds, training, hobbies, and anecdotes.

4. While all this is going on, you will still need to minimize any negative impact of staff diversity. We have already discussed the very real communication problems that accents, vocabulary, and appearance may create. To deal with this and still be politically correct, if you have a significant proportion of foreign-born nurses, then it may be useful if, at the end of *every* patient's first day in the hospital, an ombudsman visits and asks whether the patient has experienced any problems understanding what your nurses or doctors have said. By asking this of every patient, regardless of whether his or her nurses were foreign-born, you avoid stigmatizing any nurse or ethnic group. It is possible that even a standard English–speaking nurse may have accent, pronunciation, or behavioral habits that impede patient understanding. And some patients have difficulty understanding instructions or explanations no matter who is giving them.

5. If you have a diverse staff, then play on it. *You* have to convince your patients that someone who does not look and talk like them is competent and caring. Preempt the patient's perception. Display your diversity proudly around the hospital. Post group photos of your nurses, each displaying staff diversity, in your hallways. Make a collage of photos for each nursing unit and hang it in every patient room. This tells patients that you view all your nurses as constituting a valued team.

CONCLUSIONS

Because concepts of health and healing play such a key role in all nations and cultures, it is to be expected that all patients will bring their beliefs and practices with them to the hospital. Again, because of their impact on roles, personal identities, physical comfort—and survival itself—sickness and healing beliefs are typically accompanied by many nonmedical protocols that govern appropriate behaviors with and around sick people. To patients, every experience in the hospital is care and cure related. A sight, sound, meal, word, touch, or gesture that insults the patient or family may have equal or greater weight than direct (technical) acts of care in generating overall satisfaction with the clinical experience.

All patients—American-born or not—bring this baggage with them to the hospital. To nurses, physicians, and technologists—who tend to be recruited from the middle class—patients with different regional or economic backgrounds may appear to be no less culturally exotic than patients from distinct national ethnic groups. Cultural diversity has many roots. Thus, every patient must be approached as a potential bearer of a variant system of treatment and interpersonal needs.

This is why an effective program that deals with cultural diversity goes far beyond the establishment of interpreter services. Continual staff training in the beliefs, practices, and treatment expectations of different patient constituencies is essential. Both ethnic patients and staff can be pressed into service as culture brokers to mediate between the culture of the patient and the culture of the clinic.

At the same time, growing cultural diversity among staff, especially nurses, can create problems of communication with patients and colleagues. Both American- and foreign-trained nurses need to be educated about the other's role expectations and interpersonal behavioral protocols, such as interacting with authority figures or colleagues of opposite sex. By publicly celebrating its staff diversity, a hospital controls the spin about the role, acceptability, and value of its foreign staff.

ACTION FOR SATISFACTION

1. In addition to your official cadre of interpreters, identify all foreign language–speaking staff in your hospital and create a roster of potential interpreters.
2. When possible, utilize older interpreters.
3. Develop brochures in various languages to deal with various diseases. Patients can take them home and study them at leisure.

4. Assign mentors to new foreign nurses.
5. Arrange in-service workshops for all staff—not just nurses—on health beliefs of different national groups.

   If a nearby university has a medical anthropologist on staff, then by all means bring him or her in to speak on the medical beliefs of local ethnic groups. You may even wish to bring in a medical anthropologist from outside your area to speak to your staff. You can also get a reference from the head of the Society for Medical Anthropology (www.medanthro.net).

   Bring in local ethnic community representatives to talk to your staff. Ideally, get a physician and nurse who are members of the ethnic group(s) to speak. All staff, from top executives to housekeepers to volunteers, must attend. The presenters will likely not be able to give unlimited time, and you will want small groups to facilitate discussion—therefore, videotape the presentations.

   Your translators must attend the presentations and discussions. Shared ethnicity does not mean that all possess the same values and behavioral patterns. Your translators may speak the language, but they may also be second generation and unaware of beliefs and practices common to many in their own ethnic group.
6. Train former patients to counsel fellow ethnics suffering from or facing similar issues. Their role, of course, involves advocacy of appropriate treatment and importance of compliance—but not medical advice.
7. Celebrate your staff diversity in ways visible to both patients and staff. This suggests you approve of it—not just tolerate it.

REFERENCES

Betancourt, J., A. Green, and E. Carrillo. 2002. *Cultural Competence in Healthcare: Emerging Frameworks and Practical Approaches*. Field report. New York: The Commonwealth Fund.

Lewis, O. 1959. *Five Families: Mexican Case Studies in the Culture of Poverty*. N.Y: Basic Books.

Mills-Senn, P. 2005. "Avoiding Culture Clash." *Hospitals and Health Networks* 79 (4): 30–32.

Pachter, L. M. 1994. "Culture and Clinical Care: Folk Illness Beliefs and Behaviors and Their Implications for Health Care Delivery." *JAMA* 271 (9): 690–694.

SELECTED RESOURCES

These materials for your library offer specific descriptions of health beliefs and practices of various ethnic groups and suggestions on how to handle them, in addition to insight to issues of nurse diversity.

Andrews, M. M., J. S. Boyle, and T. J. Carr (eds.). 2002. *Transcultural Concepts in Nursing Care*, 4th edition. Philadelphia, PA: Lippincott, Williams & Wilkins.

D'Avanzo, C. E., and E. M. Geissler. 2004. *Pocket Guide to Cultural Assessment*, 3rd edition. St. Louis, MO: Mosby.

Dobson, S. M. 1991. *Transcultural Nursing: A Contemporary Imperative*. London: Scutari Press.

Galanti, G. 2005. *65 Tips for Foreign Born Nurses Working in American Hospitals*. SupportForNurses.com. [Online article; retrieved 1/24/05.] http://www.supportfornurses.com/products/item7.cfm.

Galanti, G. 2004. *Caring for Patients from Different Cultures*, 3rd edition. Philadelphia: University of Pennsylvania Press.

Giger, J. N, and R. E. Davidhizar (eds.). 2004. *Transcultural Nursing: Assessment and Intervention*, 4th edition. St. Louis, MO: Mosby.

Gropper, R. C. 1996. *Culture and the Clinical Encounter: An Intercultural Sensitizer for Health Professions*. Yarmouth, ME: Intercultural Press.

Harwood, A. 1981. *Ethnicity and Medical Care*. Cambridge, MA: Harvard University Press.

Lipson, J. G., S. L. Dibble, and P. A. Minarik. 1996. *Culture and Nursing Care: A Pocket Guide*. San Francisco: University of California at San Francisco Press.

Purnell, L. D., and B. J. Paulanka. 2003. *Transcultural Health Care: A Culturally Competent Approach*, 2nd edition. Philadelphia, PA: F. A. Davis.

Rundle, A., M. Carvalho, and M. Robinson (eds.). 1999. *Cultural Competence in Healthcare: A Practical Guide*. San Francisco, Jossey-Bass.

Spector, R. E. 2004. *Cultural Diversity in Health and Illness*. Upper Saddle River, NJ: Pearson Prentice Hall.

University of Washington Medical Center. Culture Clues. [Online information; retrieved 8/15/05.] http://depts.washington.edu/pfes/cultureclues.html.

Several journals also focus on diversity in healthcare. Among them are:

Holistic Nursing Practice
Journal of Cultural Diversity
Journal of Multicultural Nursing and Health

In addition, the Institute for Diversity in Health Management (an AHA affiliate) offers information on mentoring and other diversity resources on their website at www.diversityconnection.org.

CHAPTER 6

From Theory to Method:
Using Your Survey Data Effectively

To IMPROVE PATIENT satisfaction, it has to be effectively monitored. As should be clear from our earlier discussions, patient satisfaction measurement is not typical market research. All things being equal, patients do not want to use your services—ever. And the roots of patient satisfaction are far from simplistic.

You are probably already measuring patient satisfaction. In this chapter, we are concerned with making sure you use the survey data effectively. Your data reports may not look exactly like the examples that follow, but the principles of data mining are valid across all surveys.

Because patient satisfaction is important, it has to be monitored, and others beside yourself will be monitoring your patients' satisfaction. An increasing number of state hospital associations are making public the results of sporadic surveys sent to the patients of member institutions. Business/purchasing coalitions have done the same, and they are using the data to influence contracts with providers. CMS has developed the HCAHPS, a patient satisfaction survey that it expects hospitals to use for public reporting.

These report cards will increase in frequency, and you must do your homework to get good grades on them. You must measure patient satisfaction on a continuous basis and respond effectively to the data. Regardless of the survey instrument you employ, the data must be useable for improvement efforts.

POSSIBILITIES AND LIMITATIONS OF SATISFACTION SURVEYS

You must be able to break your data down by the sources of care, including nursing units, departments, medical specialties, shifts, and individual physicians. Furthermore, you must be able to analyze all these data by various patient characteristics such as age, sex, diagnosis-related group (DRG), or first-timer versus repeat patient.

Do not let anyone fool you by claiming that satisfaction survey data will solve your problems by themselves—they cannot. Survey data are limited by the number of questions you want to ask. Ask too few, and you will not get sufficient information; ask too many, and you cut the return rate substantially.

Each patient in your institution experiences thousands of interactions with your people, equipment, and physical plant. You cannot ask questions about each experience. Take admitting, for example. You could easily ask about chair comfort, privacy, courtesy, friendliness (quite different from courtesy), knowledge, speed, accuracy, and redundancy (e.g., "Did we ask you the same domestic and financial questions while registering this time that we asked you the last time you were here?"). You could ask about lighting, lobby noise, introductions, explanations, directions to rooms, and expressions of concern. You could ask 20 more questions about admitting alone, but by that time, the patient will have tossed the survey into the garbage can.

The surveys cannot identify root causes of problems. Let's say you get low scores on the courtesy of the person who admitted the patient. This is an important issue. But can you identify its underlying cause? As we noted, you cannot ask everything. Perhaps the low courtesy score is caused by a high census. Perhaps the admitting clerk is forced to answer phones and cannot pay continuous attention to the people being admitted. Perhaps the physical layout of the admitting desk makes it appear like a bank lobby and too impersonal or intimidating. Perhaps the admitting clerk is new and unsure. Perhaps the clerk has an attitude toward Medicaid or certain minority patients.

You cannot ask patients everything; even if you could, their answers still would not necessarily reveal underlying causes. A low score on the nurse's response to the call button, might have any number of possible causes—none of which are obvious to the patient. Is the problem the call light location and visibility in the nursing station? A high census? Understaffing? Mechanical failure? Is it callous nurses? Is it pesky, demanding patients who have been labeled and are being "punished" by nurses who wait just a bit longer before responding to the call? Is the call button designed to prevent electrical contact when pressed in a particular manner? All the patient knows is that she has pushed it, and no one responds. Here again, a low score tells you only that you have a particular problem—*it is up to you to dig deeper into the issue to discover the underlying cause.* No survey can do more than identify the existence and intensity of a problem. Staff have to follow through with cause identification and problem-solving techniques.

WHAT ARE PATIENT SATISFACTION SURVEYS REALLY MEASURING?

Satisfaction surveys capture patients' recollections and perceptions of care. Recollections and perceptions may not necessarily correspond with events as they actually happened. In a large sense, the issue of reality is quite unimportant. With patient satisfaction, reality is in the eye of the patient, not the provider or the person writing or reading the survey.

Even if the patient is asked an outright question about whether an event occurred (answerable by "yes" or "no"), the response reflects a subjective recollection, not necessarily reality. I recall a colleague reporting on a study of informed consent at a hospital. The interactions between surgeons and their patients were videotaped. Following surgery and recovery, patients were asked whether they had been given information about the procedure and potentially negative outcomes. Many patients who claimed not to have been given information prior to surgery actually had received such information. The researchers concluded that it was the quality of the interaction (e.g., friendliness, receptivity to questions, not appearing rushed) with the physician that governed the quantity of technical information remembered.

If a simple yes/no question can yield subjective responses, then questions offering a scale of answers provide even more opportunity for subjective judgment by the patient. If the patient is given a choice of four possible responses (i.e., "never," "almost never," "usually," and "always") to the question "How often did the nurse respond within five minutes of your pushing the call button?" then what is being elicited are perceptions, impressions, and evaluations—not an account of real events. Nurses could always respond to the call button within five minutes, and you would still have a full range of responses to the "how often . . ." question. A patient who was in pain, anxious, frightened, bored, impatient, or cantankerous might respond with "never." A patient who was well informed, comfortable, and trusting of the staff might respond with "always," even though response time might have been as high as 15 minutes.

Again, and I cannot stress this enough, if you have a low score for response time to the call button, then this does not necessarily mean you have a time problem. It could easily be a communication problem.

Patient satisfaction is indeed subjective. If someone promises you that his or her survey gets at what *really* happens in your hospital—don't believe it. All surveys tap perceptions—call them impressions, or ratings, or whatever you wish—not objective reality. These perceptions create the patient's reality. Because the whole goal of patient satisfaction measurement is to elicit the *patient's* evaluation of care rather than the provider's, the issue of accuracy is irrelevant. If patients think a wait is too long, a room too blah, a shot too painful, an explanation too obtuse, then it is. Are you going to say, "Hey, these patients are nuts! Ignore them!"? Regardless of their accuracy, you have to address these issues or your patients will continue to be dissatisfied and disloyal. If survey results show that your patients are dissatisfied, then you have a very real problem.

Survey Data Basics

You do not need fancy statistical analyses to have useful patient satisfaction data. The simplest, most basic calculations can be the basis of an effective quality improvement (QI) program.

I do not want to make analysis and reporting of satisfaction data sound too simple. It does not matter how simple or complex your data analyses are; if you do not use them, then the data are worthless. You can do multiple regression, Chronbach Alphas, and any other fancy statistical manipulation you want. If survey results are taken seriously and are responded to, then the simplest mean scores and trend charts can be a powerful tool for quality maintenance and improvement.

You must be able to break your data down by nursing unit, department, medical specialty, and product line such as cardiac cath lab. For the ED, you will want shift breakdowns as well. Although care does involve a system of processes that crosscut departments and units, care is managed, supervised, and effectively controlled by the separate administrative entities. Thus, data by unit and department are essential for QI efforts.

Ultimately, you will want to use a form of patient ID numbers to break your data down by individual physician, DRG, patient costs and charges, and so forth. In the meantime, if you know the following and respond effectively, then you can achieve high levels of patient satisfaction:

1. How are we doing overall? What does our trend look like?
2. What is scoring highest, and what is scoring lowest? Units, medical specialties, and so forth with the highest mean scores are for benchmarking and rewarding. Those with lowest scores need fixing. (A caveat here—compare comparable elements such as nursing unit to nursing unit, or physician to physician. You cannot compare nursing scores with dietary scores; dietary will always be the loser.)
3. What has changed and what has not since the last measure? A simple glance at mean scores can tell you this. In addition to looking for trends in your overall score, you need your data broken down by individual question, nursing unit, department (e.g., housekeeping, dietary, radiology), medical specialty, and key processes (e.g., discharge and continuity of care arrangements, interaction with family).
4. Is the change meaningful? You can expect some variation in your data from period to period—this is normal. If a score for a survey item or nursing unit, for example, falls within one standard deviation of the mean, then it does not differ so significantly from the mean that action is required. If a change in score clearly continues on a trend upward or downward, albeit in small increments, then it is probably meaningful. You do not need fancy statistics to tell you what your eyes can see over a period of time. On the other hand, a change may be unexpected and trend-breaking. Here, statistical significance tests can tell you if the change is also meaningful. Can you think of any reason why the score has changed? Construction? High census? Labor dispute? Bad publicity? Reorganization of some kind? If you can find a general cause, then you can then dig deeper to find root causes that will direct you to effective interventions.

5. What issues should get priority attention? Some issues are more closely linked with overall satisfaction than are others. Here, you need a simple correlation coefficient. You will want to see how strongly each question correlates with overall satisfaction. For the overall satisfaction score, you can use either your overall institution mean score, which is the mean for all the items on your survey, or the mean score of a single global question (e.g., "Please rate the overall care you received at our hospital"). The more highly correlated the item with overall satisfaction, the more important the item. If such an item has a relatively low score, then it could be having a particularly negative effect on overall patient satisfaction with care. Thus, of two items with relatively low scores, focus attention on the one more highly correlated with overall satisfaction.

6. How well do we perform *vis a vis* peers? You need access to comparative data to measure this. In addition to broad national information, you will need to compare your scores with those of various types of peers, identified by bed size, acuity, region, state, and so forth. Comparative scores tell you how patients experience and evaluate other providers. If your scores are lower than theirs are, then it is a cue for action on your part. Almost all hospital administrators assume that their institution is high in patient satisfaction. Comparative data can confirm—or contradict—this assumption.

CALCULATING AND REPORTING SCORES

Your survey may have a four-, five-, or even ten-item answer scale. In the discussions to follow, we assume you are using a five-item answer scale, with one being the lowest evaluation and five the highest.

When all the surveys are in, how should you calculate and report the scores? One way to analyze the data is to simply report scores by the percentage of responses under each category. For example:

very poor	poor	fair	good	very good
2%	4%	7%	26%	61%

The disadvantage to this kind of reporting is that it makes comparisons over time difficult. For example:

This period						*Last period*				
very poor	poor	fair	good	very good		very poor	poor	fair	good	very good
0%	1%	7%	50%	42%		3%	4%	1%	42%	50%

Which period shows better performance? The answer is difficult, because the meaning of the different combinations is open to interpretation. When you are comparing five different numbers over two periods, you are really juggling ten numbers. Is it better to have more high numbers or fewer low numbers? Comparisons can be confusing and ambiguous.

Another way of reporting scores is to combine the percentage of responses for the two top categories and then simply consider this the number of satisfied patients. This initially sounds logical, but it really does not work. In the example above, by combining the two top response categories, you would conclude that 92 percent of patients were satisfied in both this period and last period—thus, no change. But is this so? Note that during this period, 8 percent fewer patients rated you in the top category. By combining the two top categories, you would never see this. Moreover, by reporting only the two top categories, you would not see the numbers of truly dissatisfied patients (Drain 2001, 44). The intensity of dissatisfaction of patients who rate you in the lowest categories (ones and twos) has been found to be greater than the intensity of satisfaction felt by patients who give you fours and fives (Mittal and

Baldasare 1996). Patients want to take exceptionally good experiences for granted; they never want to experience poor care. When they receive poor care, they are more surprised and affected than when they get great care.

This is not to say that top-box analysis (i.e., focusing on the top response category) has no place in your repertoire. Marketing wisdom indicates that only customers who give you the top rating are likely to remain loyal. Thus, the percentage of fives among your respondents represents that portion of your market share you can count on keeping over the long haul. All others are at risk for defection. Your goal should be to increase the proportion of fives while reducing the numbers of ones and twos.

Top-box and bottom-box analyses are definitely helpful; however, the most useful scoring for ongoing analysis and improvement activities are mean scores that include all five response categories. This reflects the full range of patient experiences.

In analyzing your data, convert your four- or five-item response scale to a zero-to-100 scale, calculate a single mean score using all response categories, and report this single mean. This process has many advantages. First, it condenses everything into a single number that is influenced by both high and low evaluations. Second, a single number is easy to compare across departments, across time, or across hospitals. Third, most people are accustomed to being graded on a zero-to-100 scale, so the reports will make more sense to your staff. Fourth, by stretching the scale out (fours and fives on a five-point scale become 75 and 100), the score becomes more sensitive. Even reporting scores by the tenth of a point allows only 10 numbers between 4.0 and 5.0. However, 250 tenths stand between 75.0 and 100.0. To calculate mean scores on a zero-to-100 basis, you can convert a five-point scale as follows:

	very poor	poor	fair	good	very good
Scale on survey	1	2	3	4	5
Conversion	0	25	50	75	100

SCORE VARIANCE

Obviously, you will be very concerned with upward or downward change. How much change is significant? You probably already know about t-tests, standard errors, standard deviations, and so forth, and can calculate statistical significance. Of more conceptual importance is the need to recognize that patient satisfaction scores typically fall within a very narrow range. Moreover, this range is at the high end of the scale. Do not expect a huge spread in scores between departments, nursing units, physicians, or any other units of analysis. The reason is twofold. First, care these days really is good. Patients have great trust in healthcare providers and generally do believe that care is first rate. Second, as I have indicated before, patients are intimidated by healthcare and are generally reluctant to bite the hand that heals them.

Thus, contrary to what many people think, those who answer surveys are not the disgruntled complainers. Typically, 85 to 90 percent of respondents rate their care in the top two response categories. As a result, scores for most aspects of care (except food), tend to be in a fairly narrow high range. Your highest and lowest scores for individual survey items, nursing units, and so forth may be no more than 10 or 15 points apart. Nursing units, for example, might typically range from a low of 78 to a high of 93. On a 100-point scale, that is not much variance. This means that small differences in score can reflect some real differences in performance. A two-point difference between nursing units or time periods can reflect a 15 or 20 percent variance. This could be of importance when it comes to realistic goal setting.

INTERPRETING THE DATA

A brief tour through some typical satisfaction report data will illustrate their utility. These real data from real hospital reports were generated for these examples.

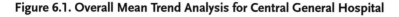

Figure 6.1. Overall Mean Trend Analysis for Central General Hospital

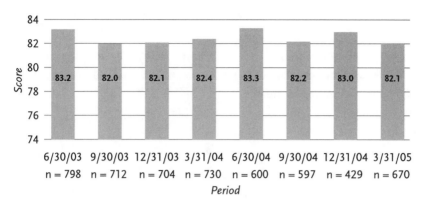

	6/30/03	9/30/03	12/31/03	3/31/04	6/30/04	9/30/04	12/31/04	3/31/05
Score	83.2	82.0	82.1	82.4	83.3	82.2	83.0	82.1
	n = 798	n = 712	n = 704	n = 730	n = 600	n = 597	n = 429	n = 670

Period

You will probably want to start off by asking, "How are we doing, overall?" Figure 6.1 shows the present overall score and its trend over eight quarters. The overall mean satisfaction score for this period is 82.1 on a zero-to-100 scale for Central General Hospital (CGH, a fictitious hospital). The score is down almost a full point from the previous quarter. Given my earlier warning that these scores tend to fall within a narrow range of only 15 to 20 points, a drop of one point from last period represents at least a 5 percent decline. What has been going on?

Looking at eight quarters of data, it is clear that CGH is going nowhere in terms of patient satisfaction. The trend is virtually flat. Of course, if CGH's scores were the top in the country, then maintaining this flat trajectory at the top of the heap would be commendable. But as we will see below, this is not the case—which is another reason why comparative data are essential.

Figure 6.2 on the following page answers the question, "What is scoring highest, and what is scoring lowest?" This simple chart lists the survey item scores from highest to lowest. To save space, we have only included the eight highest and eight lowest scoring questions. As at most hospitals, physicians and nurses tend to score high at

Figure 6.2. Central General Hospital Scores Ranked (1/1/05–3/31/05)

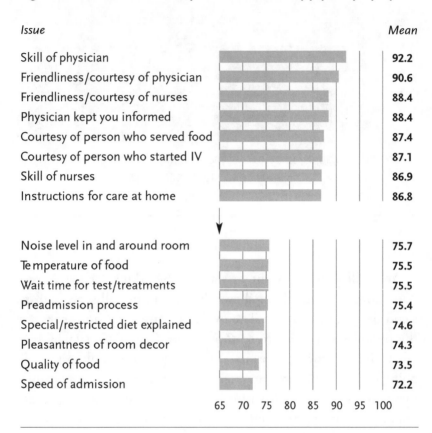

Issue	Mean
Skill of physician	92.2
Friendliness/courtesy of physician	90.6
Friendliness/courtesy of nurses	88.4
Physician kept you informed	88.4
Courtesy of person who served food	87.4
Courtesy of person who started IV	87.1
Skill of nurses	86.9
Instructions for care at home	86.8
Noise level in and around room	75.7
Temperature of food	75.5
Wait time for test/treatments	75.5
Preadmission process	75.4
Special/restricted diet explained	74.6
Pleasantness of room decor	74.3
Quality of food	73.5
Speed of admission	72.2

65 70 75 80 85 90 95 100

CGH. Typically, too, food and room issues fall at the bottom. Note that the lowest scoring issue is speed of admission.

In themselves, the scores of individual survey items are not actionable. They are useful only when compared with past performance, with external competitors, or with comparable issues on your survey. Without comparative data, you cannot really judge whether 72.2 for speed of admission is high or low. However, if this score represents a significant decline from last period, then it becomes more meaningful. Similarly, if 72.2 is ten points beneath the national average, then you have a real problem.

Figure 6.3. Central General Hospital's Greatest Increase in Scores by Issue (1/1/05–3/31/05)

Issue	Mean Last Period n = 429	Change	Mean This Period n = 670
Informing family about condition/treatment	82.8	+1.7	84.5
Courtesy of person who started IV	85.5	+1.4	86.9
Patient included in decisions about treatment	81.9	+1.3	83.2
Skill of person who started IV	80.4	+1.2	81.6
Physician kept you informed	86.3	+1.1	87.4

Within any section of the survey, there should be consistency. For example, nursing activities rated by patients include demeanor, information, skill, empathy, promptness, and response to being called. All of these constitute key elements in nursing performance. All should be performed at or near the same level of quality. If the score for courtesy of nursing staff is five or six points lower than most other nurse items, then this is anomalous and should be investigated.

Figure 6.3 indicates items increasing the most. What has gone up the most from last quarter? Personnel responsible for these five issues deserve kudos this quarter. These results should be posted.

Figure 6.4 on the following page demonstrates the items declining the most. This list is headed by speed of admission, which is down by a whopping 3.9 points from last quarter. The decline is significant at the .05 level. What has happened? An increased census? A procedural change? Construction? Personnel issues (e.g., moral problems, high staff turnover)?

Also significantly lower are three accommodation-related issues —noise, room temperature, and pleasantness of room decor. Check these scores by nursing unit to see if you can pinpoint the cause. Are

Figure 6.4. Central General Hospital's Greatest Decrease in Scores by Issue (1/1/05–3/31/05)

Issue	Mean Last Period n = 429	Change	Mean This Period n = 670
Speed of admission	76.1	−3.9	72.2
Noise level in and around room	78.9	−3.2	75.7
Room temperature	79.2	−2.7	76.5
Pleasantness of room decor	76.0	−1.7	74.3
Patient felt ready for discharge	84.4	−1.6	82.8

these low scores hospital-wide, or are they limited to a specific nursing unit or area? If the low scores are not caused by construction, then get nursing and maintenance together to brainstorm.

The decline in the extent to which the patient felt ready to be discharged from the hospital is likely a result of information failure, not physical condition of the patient per se. Another item in the discharge section of the survey, the adequacy of instructions for caring for yourself at home (not shown here), declined by half a point. However, this small drop probably does not fully account for the larger decline in readiness for discharge. Patients were likely not given adequate information upon admission about expected length of stay or explanations about their condition and prognosis at the time of discharge, and they felt less at ease about leaving the hospital's protective environment.

Figure 6.5 compares and ranks nursing units. Pretty much everything happens to patients via their nursing units. Even admitting is related to the medical specialty of the unit, bed availability on the unit, signage, and so forth. Radiological exams may occur elsewhere in the hospital, but the experience is also linked to the unit through medical specialty, transport, and so forth. Food scores may vary

Figure 6.5. Central General Hospital Nursing Units Ranked (All Issues)

Unit	Mean 10/1/04–12/31/04	Mean 1/1/05–3/31/05	Change
4S	86.0	86.7	+0.7
4W	82.6	83.9	+1.3
3E	83.8	82.5	−1.3
3S	79.9	82.2	+2.3
4N	81.7	80.2	−1.5
4E	81.0	79.3	−1.7
3W	82.9	78.9	−4.0

from unit to unit depending on such things as location and nurse protocols for tray distribution, among others.

In the figure, the units are ranked from highest to lowest overall mean score, with all items on the survey contributing to the mean. We note that 3W is not only the lowest scoring unit, but is also down a whopping four points from last period. What is going on? Before looking at specific issues that may be behind 3W's low scores, look at the trend.

Figure 6.6 on the following page is a trend analysis of nursing unit 3W. The precipitous decline on 3W of four points is not part of an ongoing trend. Indeed, by looking back eight quarters, we see a general trend upwards with some peaks and valleys. This suggests that the recent dip is situational rather than typical and should be responded to with this in mind. Something very unusual must have happened to trigger such a sharp drop in one quarter. No one survey issue or even section of the survey, such as nursing or dietary, can account for the large drop in 3W's score this period. Forty-eight items contribute toward each nursing unit's overall score. This suggests that something major happening on 3W is affecting a wide range of patient experiences on that unit.

Figure 6.6. Mean Trend Analysis for Nursing Unit 3W

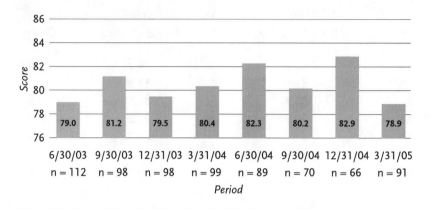

	6/30/03	9/30/03	12/31/03	3/31/04	6/30/04	9/30/04	12/31/04	3/31/05
Score	79.0	81.2	79.5	80.4	82.3	80.2	82.9	78.9
	n = 112	n = 98	n = 98	n = 99	n = 89	n = 70	n = 66	n = 91

Period

We can get some insight by looking at specific sections of the survey by nursing unit. We will look at two sections here: nursing and accommodations.

Figure 6.7 lists the scores for individual issues that make up the nursing section of the survey. The lowest score for each issue is in bold italic type. Why is 3W's score for nurse response to the call button so low? Both 3W and 4N, as well as 4E, have unusually low scores for nurse attention to patients' personal or special needs and nurse attitudes toward special requests, plus keeping patients informed. These are key interactional issues. Not surprisingly, patients also judge their general skills to be lower. What characteristics (e.g., staffing, census, physical plant) do these nursing units share? 4N is clearly not doing as well as other units on the core nursing issues. What is happening? 4N can use some attention.

Let's see whether we can focus in on the low room/accommodation scores. In Figure 6.8, the room items are broken down by nursing unit. Patients clearly do not like unit 3W, but a number of others are also low scoring. Check 3W's room scores for the last period. Is there some construction going on? Is it a particularly old unit? Why are 3W and 4N so low for room decor? Why, for that matter, is 4W so high for room decor? Is it recently remodeled?

Figure 6.7. Nursing Issues by Unit (1/1/05–3/31/05)

	3S	3E	3W	4S	4E	4W	4N
Friendliness/courtesy of nurses	92.3	90.0	84.8	92.7	85.8	87.7	*84.4*
Promptness of response to call	83.2	85.5	*74.4*	87.2	80.0	84.8	79.9
Nurses' attitude toward requests	90.1	88.0	81.6	89.7	83.3	86.1	*81.1*
Attention special/personal needs	87.3	86.0	*79.8*	88.9	80.7	85.8	80.1
Nurses kept you informed	85.4	84.8	78.8	87.2	80.8	84.2	*76.5*
Skill of the nurses	90.9	88.8	83.6	90.0	84.5	87.3	*82.1*

Note: Lowest score for each issue in bold italic type.

Figure 6.8. Room/Accommodations by Nursing Unit (1/1/05–3/31/05)

	3S	3E	3W	4S	4E	4W	4N
Mean for Room Issues	*79.0*	*77.8*	*75.4*	*81.6*	*78.0*	*82.1*	*76.6*
Pleasantness of room decor	75.9	73.7	69.4	75.6	78.1	83.2	*69.1*
Room cleanliness	80.1	76.8	*72.5*	81.0	77.7	81.2	75.5
Courtesy of person cleaning room	85.9	84.1	*81.9*	87.8	84.2	88.2	82.2
Room temperature	73.2	77.1	77.2	77.3	*73.0*	77.9	77.8
Noise level in and around room	78.3	74.7	*72.5*	80.0	74.6	76.2	73.8
TV call button, etc., worked	81.5	82.5	*80.7*	88.2	81.6	85.8	82.9

Note: Lowest score for each issue in bold italic type.

Are there more windows, or is the view better? Here, high scoring units could offer clues to best practices for other units. Why would patients on 3W complain about cleanliness so much? Why do they think so little of cleaning staff courtesy?

Not every item is of equal importance to patient satisfaction; you need to know what to focus on. As indicated above, score itself does not give you all the information. You need to know how each item is related to overall satisfaction. This allows you to "weight" each survey item. Correlation coefficients for the

Figure 6.9. Survey Items Ranked by Correlation with Overall Satisfaction

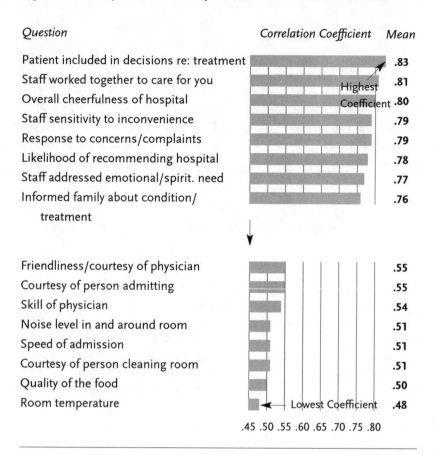

Question	Correlation Coefficient	Mean
Patient included in decisions re: treatment		.83
Staff worked together to care for you	Highest	.81
Overall cheerfulness of hospital	Coefficient	.80
Staff sensitivity to inconvenience		.79
Response to concerns/complaints		.79
Likelihood of recommending hospital		.78
Staff addressed emotional/spirit. need		.77
Informed family about condition/ treatment		.76
Friendliness/courtesy of physician		.55
Courtesy of person admitting		.55
Skill of physician		.54
Noise level in and around room		.51
Speed of admission		.51
Courtesy of person cleaning room		.51
Quality of the food		.50
Room temperature	Lowest Coefficient	.48

.45 .50 .55 .60 .65 .70 .75 .80

relationship between each survey item and overall patient satisfaction with care are calculated in Figure 6.9. Here, the mean for each item is correlated with the overall mean of the survey. The higher the correlation, the more likely that the score for that item and the overall mean score go up or down together. More highly correlated issues can have a greater impact—positive or negative—on overall satisfaction. Figure 6.9 presents only the eight items (out of a total of 48) most correlated and the eight items least correlated with overall patient satisfaction at CGH.

All items on the survey are and should be correlated significantly with the overall satisfaction score. Even the item least correlated with overall satisfaction—room temperature—has a coefficient of .48, which is sizable. Room temperature does have an effect on the patient's overall evaluation of care. This effect, however, is far less than that of other aspects of care.

The issue of greatest potential importance to CGH patients— most highly correlated with overall satisfaction—is the issue of patients being included in the planning of their care. Patients respond positively to such empowerment. Patients also feel that coordination of care is very important. With so many staff members coming, going, and performing myriad tasks, patients want to know that each is aware of what the others have done or learned.

If the items most highly correlated with satisfaction are also high scoring, then they can have a major positive impact on overall satisfaction. If they are low scoring, then they can have a major negative impact on patients' evaluation of care.

On the other hand, items least correlated with overall satisfaction have less theoretical effect on it. We have already noted that speed of admission is the lowest scoring item on CGH's survey and is also the item declining the most from the last period. However, the low, falling score must be balanced against the fact that speed of admission is one of the items least correlated with overall satisfaction. Thus, it may not be a high priority for change. Of far higher priority should be issues that score low and are also highly correlated with overall satisfaction.

Figure 6.10 on the following page links both correlation and score to create a priority index. Remember that correlation coefficients are not satisfaction scores. Items highly correlated with overall patient satisfaction can be either high or low scoring. Items that are more highly correlated with overall satisfaction and are also lower scoring have potentially greater negative impact on satisfaction and should get higher priority for allocation of attention and resources.

This figure is very useful and simply created. Rank questions by score, giving highest weight to items with the lowest scores. Then,

Figure 6.10. Priority Index for Central General Hospital (1/1/05–3/31/05)

Rank	Quarters in Top Ten	Question	Mean Score (Weight)	Correlation Coefficient (Weight)	Priority Index (Combined Weights)
1	6	Response to concerns/complaints	81.5 (35)	.79 (43)	35 / 43 — 78
2	3	Staff addressed emotional/spirit. need	81.1 (37)	.77 (40)	37 / 40 — 77
3	1	Staff sensitivity to inconvenience	82.3 (31)	.79 (44)	31 / 44 — 75
4	2	Patient included in treatment decisions	83.2 (25)	.83 (48)	25 / 48 — 73
5	4	Overall cheerfulness of hospital	83.4 (24)	.80 (45)	24 / 45 — 69
6	4	Nurses kept you informed	82.8 (28)	.76 (39)	28 / 39 — 67
7	1	Temperature of the food	75.5 (42)	.63 (28)	42 / 28 — 66
8	1	Wait time for test/treatments	75.5 (43)	.62 (22)	43 / 22 — 65
9	3	Special/restricted diet explained	74.6 (45)	.60 (19)	45 / 19 — 64
10	5	Staff concern for privacy	83.1 (26)	.76 (37)	26 / 37 — 63
44		Courtesy of person admitting	85.4 (13)	.55 (7)	13 / 7 — 20
45		Courtesy of person cleaning room	84.7 (17)	.51 (3)	17 / 3 — 20
46		Courtesy of person who served food	87.1 (6)	.56 (10)	6 / 10 — 16
47		Friendliness/courtesy of physician	90.6 (2)	.55 (8)	2 / 8 — 10
48		Skill of physician	92.2 (1)	.54 (6)	1 / 6 — 7

rank questions by correlation coefficient, giving highest weight to items most highly correlated with overall satisfaction. Finally, add the two weights to get your priority index. Higher priority index numbers represent issues with more potential negative impact on your patients' overall evaluation of care. Attention to these issues should give you more "bang for your buck."

Forty-eight questions compose the CGH survey. The issue with the lowest score is assigned a weight of 48, the issue with second lowest score a 47, and so forth. The issue with the highest mean score is assigned the lowest weight of one. For the correlation co-efficients, the issue with highest correlation coefficient is assigned a weight of 48, the issue with second highest coefficient gets a 47, and so forth. For each question, the two weights for its score and correlation coefficient are added together to get its priority rank. Score and correlation with satisfaction are distinct, unrelated factors. Therefore, the item with highest priority may not be the item with the lowest score or highest correlation. The highest priority issue reflects a combination of dissatisfaction and importance sufficient to have the most potential negative impact on the patient's overall experience of care. At the same time, by improving these issues you have the greatest potential positive impact on your patients. In this example, we see the ten items that top CGH's priority index, plus the five lowest; these latter are included simply to give you an idea of what is typically of lowest priority.

Heading the priority list is the issue of service recovery—how well staff respond to patients' problems and complaints. This item has the fifth highest correlation coefficient (weight of 43 out of 48) and a sufficiently low score (weight of 35 out of 48). 35 + 43 = 78. Therefore, it has a potentially significant negative influence on CGH patients' evaluation of care. The second item at the top of the priority index is satisfaction with chaplain services. This is rather unusual. Nationally, chaplain issues are usually of less importance and relatively high scoring. Does CGH have a particularly church-oriented or religiously conservative patient constituency? Is the chaplain doing something that is particularly unsettling to patients? Are staff creating expectations about chaplain services that the hospital cannot meet? (Note: As we will discuss in a subsequent chapter, survey numbers can identify the existence of a problem and generally point to general sources. They cannot usually pinpoint the specific cause—that's up to you.).

The third issue at the top of the priority index is the staff's sensitivity to the problems and inconveniences that sickness and hospitalization can cause. This issue is a direct reflection of a key element of illness discussed in a previous chapter—the threats to role and identity caused by sickness and hospitalization. CGH's patients apparently feel threatened and perceive that they are not getting sufficient support (e.g., empathy, sick-role accommodation) from staff.

A final piece of information from this chart: For how many periods has each issue been among the top ten in the priority index? This provides insight into QI progress since the previous data period. Notice that the lead issue, staff response to concerns or complaints, has been a top-ten priority for six consecutive periods. Essentially, this suggests that CGH has not done much to address the service recovery issue effectively. Maybe nothing has been done at all! Is this the case?

If you can tap into an outside source for comparative data, then so much the better. While internal data are essential for monitoring performance over time, they tell you nothing about the relative quality of the care you deliver. For example, your overall nursing score may be 93 on a 100-point scale, and you may worry that it is not higher. You may want to implement programs for further improvement. What you do not know is that your 93 might place you at or near the very top of hospital nursing scores nationally, meaning that you are already great. In this case, a program directed at improving patient satisfaction with nursing would not be a wise use of QI resources, and it might have a negative impact on nurse morale.

Figure 6.11 displays the survey section scores for CGH. If CGH had no comparative data, then administration might naturally focus

Figure 6.11. Survey Section Scores (n = 684, 1/1/05–3/31/05)

Section	Mean This Period	Peer Group Mean Score	Percentile Rank Within Peer Group
Admissions	87.3	86.4	56
Nursing	**85.7**	**88.2**	**22**
Personal Issues	85.8	88.0	37
Visitors and Family	85.3	87.2	39
Physician	85.1	86.0	43
Discharge	84.6	84.4	52
Tests and Treatments	83.1	85.0	34
Room/Accomodations	81.8	77.1	88
Dietary	**79.8**	**76.2**	**80**

on dietary's score of 79.8 as the lowest of its departments. It is six points below nursing. In truth, CGH would be wasting its efforts and resources because dietary is in the 80th percentile in its national comparative database. That is good, solid performance. Nursing, on the other hand, falls in the 22nd percentile, meaning that 78 percent of database hospitals have higher satisfaction scores for nursing than CGH. Here, comparative data indicate that CGH's real patient satisfaction problem lies with nursing, not food. Because nursing contributes far more than does food to the patient's overall evaluation of care (much higher correlation coefficients), both the potential negative impact and the opportunity for significant overall improvement are magnified.

The more peer institutions you can compare yourself against, the more precise and realistic your evaluation of your own performance can be. If you are a small hospital in a modest-size community, then your effect on patients is not the same as that of a large, urban teaching institution. On average, larger hospitals score lower than smaller. Teaching hospitals score lower than non-teaching hospitals. On average, hospitals in large cities score lower than hospitals in smaller communities. Larger hospitals in larger towns have to work harder to satisfy patients. The more peer performance information you have, the more realistic will be your understanding of how you are doing.

CONCLUSIONS

As suggested earlier, some very basic data breakdowns and statistics will give you a diamond mine of information and insight. Constant review of your satisfaction data will sensitize you to changes and trends. Remember to compare apples to apples. When using internal data to note what is scoring highest and what is scoring lowest, don't look across specialties or departments. Nursing and food are not comparable. Focus instead on which nursing unit is highest or lowest, or on which nursing item on the survey is highest or lowest.

You can compare nursing and food when you take external peer data into account. Percentile rank among peers is a good indicator of relative performance among your departments. If nursing is in the 20th percentile nationally and your dietary is in the 80th percentile, then dietary is performing better than nursing, regardless of the raw scores.

Of course, you want data that are statistically valid. But another form of validity is your own recognition of the truth in the numbers. Do the scores make sense? If a score goes down and you know why, then you do not need statistics to tell you that what you are seeing is real. Sometimes staff attempt to cast doubt on the validity of patient satisfaction scores—particularly when their own scores are the ones that are low!

ACTION FOR SATISFACTION

1. Look at the obvious numbers first. What are the largest increases or decreases in score from the previous period? Investigate these

issues. It is usually easier to identify the reasons behind larger changes. Such a detection exercise promotes confidence in your survey, as it demonstrates that the survey is sensitive enough to pick up on changes in procedures or circumstances. Your staff need to have confidence in the survey if they are to respond seriously and effectively to the data.

2. Look for trends in your data. Sometimes small changes from one period to the next are not statistically significant. But regular movement up or down can reveal meaningful change.

3. Use correlation coefficients and a priority index to identify appropriate targets for improvement. Issues more highly correlated with overall satisfaction have potentially more effect on the patient's overall evaluation of care. If these issues also happen to be lower scoring, then their negative impact is multiplied. Attention to these issues will give you more bang for your buck in terms of improving your overall score.

4. Get comparative data, if you can. Internal data analyses are your guide to improving performance. But you will not know whether your performance really needs improvement. If you are one of the best hospitals in the country, then your patient satisfaction strategy is essentially one of maintenance rather than improvement. Comparative data tell you whether you are in the ball park or out of it, and whether you need mere maintenance or serious repair.

REFERENCES

Drain, M. 2001. "Quality Improvement in Primary Care and the Importance of Patient Perceptions." *Journal of Ambulatory Care Management* 24 (2): 30–46.

Mittal, V., and P. M. Baldasare. 1996. "Eliminate the Negative." *Journal of Health Care Marketing* 16 (3): 24–31.

CHAPTER 7

Mining the Data for Insights

GOING BEYOND SIMPLE mean scores can get you closer to identifying key problem areas that need fixing or high performers that deserve rewards. As we have seen, you can get a lot of insight simply by looking at question means as well as unit, department, and specialty or service means. However, the deeper you go into the data, the more specific will be your understanding of what is going on. This chapter provides some examples of insights you can get by breaking down the data.

Drill deeper into the data to answer some of the following questions:

- Do different types of patients have different experiences of your care?
- Does age or sex make a difference? Does payer?
- Is care better in certain parts of your facility?
- Does care differ by season, month, day, or time (e.g., ED shift)?
- Does care differ by staff member?
- Does care differ by condition or procedure?

- Is there a relationship between satisfaction and profit for specific conditions?

Ideally, a patient identifier on the survey, such as a barcode or number, will allow you to link to patient records. With this identifier, you will be able to run satisfaction data against a host of other information about the patient. With links to records, you can run patient satisfaction against financial data (e.g., costs, charges, usage, length of stay), physician, procedure, or condition (e.g., DRG). If you do not or cannot put an identifier on the survey, then at the very least you can add a few key demographic questions that will allow you to examine patient satisfaction by sex, age, length of stay, first-time versus repeat customer, ED admit, type of insurance, and so forth.

You will need sufficient survey returns to perform an accurate analysis. For example, if you get an average of 40 returns per nursing unit, then you cannot break the data from any one unit down by a half-dozen patient age categories. With five or six cases in each age category, the data would not be statistically valid. However, with 500 or 600 returns for the whole hospital, most issues and departments will have been experienced and evaluated by most respondents. You can easily break down individual questions or survey sections by a half-dozen age categories and get good, valid data.

ANALYSIS BY LENGTH OF STAY

Simple data slicing can give you a lot of useful information. The head of CGH's food service wants to improve scores. In Figure 7.1, the food items on the survey are sliced by length of stay of respondents. By and large, the shorter the stay, the less that patients like the food service. In particular, patients in for a day or less feel they have little choice of meals because menus are usually handed out on the previous day. As day surgery grows in frequency, short stays may be increasing. Providing a varied menu for same-day or

**Figure 7.1. Means for Food Service Items by Length of Stay
(1/1/05–3/31/05)**

	1 day	2–3 days	4–5 days	6–10 days	11+ days
Information diet	75.2	77.8	78.4	80.6	79.2
Temperature of the food	76.3	76.1	75.9	77.7	76.6
Quality of the food	73.9	74.8	75.8	79.1	77.3
Received what you ordered	72.5	78.9	80.1	81.6	79.4

one-day patients may result in a significant increase in satisfaction with CGH's food.

On the other hand, note that those in for longest stays begin to find fault with the food service. This may be inevitable if your menu is on, say, a seven-day cycle. You may want to add some special touches for those patients who overlap the next repetitive meal cycle.

ANALYSIS BY AGE AND MEDICAL SPECIALTY

Here is a great example of what you can learn from drilling down into the data.

CGH had consistently low scores for skill in starting IVs, as shown in Figure 7.2 on the following page. In fact, CGH's latest score of 78.8 for IV starts puts them in the second percentile nationally, meaning that 98 percent of hospitals in the database did better than CGH. Patient satisfaction with IV starts was fully ten points below the hospital's mean for all other survey items.

CGH's management was very unhappy with these data. Initially, they assumed this was a technical issue and were ready to implement a costly retraining program for all IV personnel. Before embarking on this, however, the survey administrator decided to look at their satisfaction data more deeply. Management decided to test whether

Figure 7.2. Skill of IV Starter

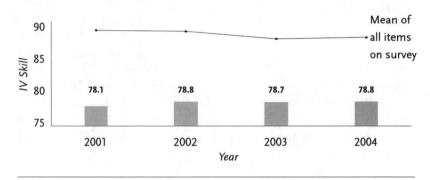

Figure 7.3. Skill of IV Starter by Patient Age

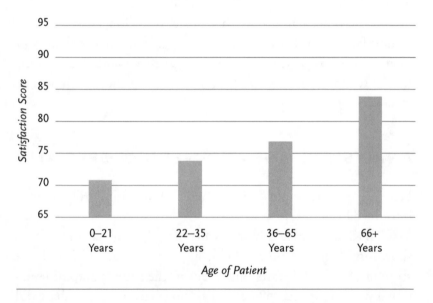

the ratings were age related. Figure 7.3 demonstrates that older patients' satisfaction with IV starts is well within the national average.
Younger patients at CGH clearly do not like their IV starts. It makes
no sense to believe that the same staff use different levels of skill with
older and younger patients. Rather, older patients are likely more
familiar with IVs than younger ones. Therefore, younger patients

Figure 7.4. Skill in Starting IV by Age Group and Specialty

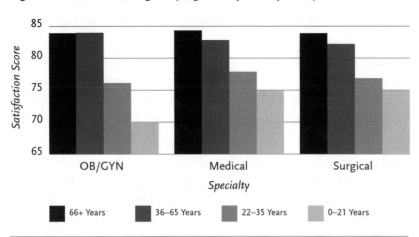

need more explanations about what IVs are like—where the needle goes in, how much it will or will not hurt, what keeps the needle from moving around, how the drip works, and so forth.

The result of this finding was a simple inservice discussion and short brochure for nurses, stressing information that should be given to younger or first-time patients. IV start scores soared.

As long as they were looking more deeply at IV starts, CGH's staff decided to keep on searching for insights. They sliced IV start scores by medical specialty as well as age (see Figure 7.4). As expected, all services showed a strong age component in patient evaluations of IV starts. Obstetrics and gynecology, however, exhibited the most dramatic age differential. Why?

It is a good bet that the older women are gynecological patients, and the youngest are there to deliver babies. A staff focus group revealed that obstetrics nurses harbored significant ambivalence about young, unmarried mothers. Nurses in the unit were themselves mothers, typically with teenaged daughters. Young, unwed, pregnant girls offended the nurses' moral values. Moreover, while certainly empathizing with these girls, obstetrics nurses also felt maternal frustration at the social and economic damage that young, single motherhood can do to a life. These less-than-positive feelings led to even greater reticence—and thus less information sharing—while they cared for the youngest obstetric patients. The deeper analyses of quantitative data led to a qualitative reevaluation of the obstetrics nurses' shared value system (something very unquantitative). Increased sensitivity to their own value systems led nurses in obstetrics to reshape their mode of interaction with young mothers. They might feel frustration toward some of the girls, but they could hide it better and communicate with them better. This also helped boost scores.

As I indicated earlier, satisfaction survey data are necessarily limited in specificity and usually cannot pinpoint root causes of problems. You cannot ask specific questions about every possible patient experience or cause of problems. The insights to causes underlying the IV issues above came from staff, not from the survey. Identifying the age issue did not identify the root cause. Surveys only narrow the field of analysis. The data offer a starting point for in-house discussions and problem solving.

ANALYSIS BY PAYER

Figure 7.5 breaks down the data from CGH's ED by payer. Why are patients insured by insurer #1 so much more satisfied with your ED?

Figure 7.5. Major Payers and Satisfaction in ED (1/1/05–3/31/05)

Payer	n	Satisfaction Scores
Insurer #1	61	83.3
HMO	26	81.1
Insurer #2	11	77.7
Medicare	83	76.4
Self-pay	56	76.2
Medicaid	45	75.1
Insurer #3	149	73.5

Why are patients insured by #3 so dissatisfied? Your largest group of patients is insured by company #3 (n = 149 suggests this); focus serious attention on the experience of their customers—remember, your customers are their customers. Do they share a particular demographic characteristic such as age, sex, or income? Do these patients tend to come from a single area of town, or from a particular local business' health plan? What clauses in their insurance might create payment problems that they blame on your ED?

IDENTIFYING INDIVIDUAL PHYSICIANS

Measuring ED satisfaction scores by individual physician is an example of physician profiling. With some sort of patient identifier on the survey, you can identify the physician who treated the patient. Figure 7.6 demonstrates that two of your highest-volume ED physicians are among your lowest satisfaction performers. Doctor 923 is especially worrisome. He sees more patients than any other physician, and thus his low patient-satisfaction performance has a big influence on overall ED score. Doctor 350 is the worst performer. Be a little careful in rushing to judgment, however, because 19 survey returns for this period may not provide a statistically significant score when compared with other physicians. If scuttlebutt suggests

Figure 7.6. Emergency Department Physician Profiling (1/1/05–3/31/05)

Physician Code	n	Satisfaction Scores
307	22	85.9
416	40	83.9
202	62	83.3
714	47	82.9
525	12	81.8
923	260	**78.8**
491	58	78.2
350	19	**75.6**

that Doctor 350 is indeed bad with patients, then talk the issue over with him or her and wait for the next set of scores before making an official comment or response.

USING MULTIPLE VARIABLES: PHYSICIAN, PROFIT, AND SATISFACTION

Measuring satisfaction and profit by physician allows an even more complicated and insightful analysis. Figure 7.7 looks at the medically (as opposed to surgically) treated cardiac inpatients treated by the four highest-volume attending physicians. Three variables are presented: (1) patient satisfaction with the physician, (2) patient satisfaction with the overall hospital experience, and (3) mean profit per case.

The chart is very instructive. The hospital suffers an average loss of $318 for every cardiac patient treated medically by Doctor 1. Moreover, Doctor 1 is clearly not satisfying his patients very well. At the same time, his patients are quite satisfied with the overall hospital experience. What is going on? Maybe Doctor 1 requires a much longer length of stay than other doctors for the same types of cardiac patients, and his patients like the extended care, even though they do not like him personally. Doctor 2, on the other hand, is the profit star for CGH, averaging $1,045 per patient, although her individual satisfaction scores are pretty low. Doctor 3 would appear to represent the best compromise. Patients like him, and he brings the hospital a good profit and high satisfaction scores. What personal and professional characteristics does he exhibit? Perhaps he could be used as a role model for the others. Doctor 4 is an all-around satisfaction champ, but he, too, is a money loser for the hospital. What is he doing that keeps his costs per patient high? This is a good example of how drill-down data analysis offers some specific avenues for investigation and priority setting. Let's explore the volume, profit, and satisfaction issues further.

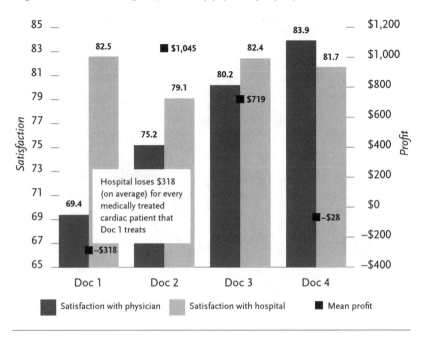

ANALYSIS BY DIAGNOSIS-RELATED GROUP (DRG)

When looking at medical versus surgical treatment of high-volume cardiac patients, imaginative graphics can give you a lot of insight. Figure 7.8 on the following page looks at four variables: (1) patient satisfaction, (2) surgical versus medical treatment, (3) profit per patient, and (4) volume of patients seen for each DRG. Profit per case runs up on the left, while satisfaction increases toward the right on the bottom. Volume is reflected in the size of the circle.

These represent CGH's highest volume DRGs. According to the figure, the biggest volume comes from medically treated heart failure and shock (DRG 127), but CGH is not making any money on

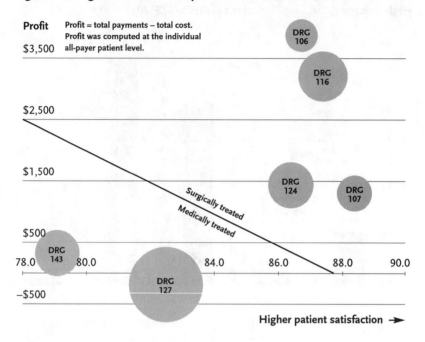

Figure 7.8. High-Volume DRGs by Profit and Patient Satisfaction

DRG 106: Coronary bypass with cardiac cath.
DRG 116: Other permanent cardiac pacemaker implant or PTCA with coronary art. st.
DRG 124: Circulatory disorders except AMI, with cardiac cath. and complex diag.
DRG 107: Coronary bypass without cardiac cath.
DRG 143: Chest pain
DRG 127: Heart failure and shock

it. Patient satisfaction, too, is quite modest. CGH has some modest profit from treating chest pain (DRG 143), but these patients are quite dissatisfied with the care.

On the other hand, all of CGH's surgically treated patients make money for the hospital. In addition, patients are far more satisfied—by at least four points—with surgical treatment than with medical treatment. CGH should look more closely at big-volume DRG 127 to see what may be affecting patient satisfaction for a large number of customers.

IDENTIFYING PRIORITY
IMPROVEMENT TARGETS

CGH's single biggest volume DRG was 127, and they are not doing a good job satisfying patients. To get more specific information about where to focus improvement efforts, look at data from surveys that were filled out by patients with DRG 127. Then, create a priority index out of all the survey questions (see Figure 6.10). Items scoring lower, but that are more highly correlated with overall satisfaction, rank higher in priority.

Figure 7.9 is the priority index for DRG 127. The first column is the combined priority index for the item. The second and third columns show the figures that go into creating the priority rank. The second column is the correlation coefficient (correlation with overall satisfaction) and the third is the mean score of the item. Figure 7.9 lists only the five issues at the top of the priority index of CGH. By focusing on these five issues, the satisfaction of patients within DRG 127 will likely be improved.

The list is headed by the issue of service recovery: "Staff response to concerns/complaints made during patient's stay." This

Figure 7.9. Priority Index for DRG 127—Top Five Issues (1/1/05–3/31/05)

	Priority Index	Corr. Coef.	Item Mean
Staff response to concerns/complaints made during patient's stay	98	.91	72.0
Staff effort to include patient in decisions about treatment	96	.89	73.1
Physician's concern for patient's questions and worries	94	.86	81.0
Time physician spent with patient	90	.82	78.7
Information given to family about condition/treatment	88	.86	82.1

item potentially has the biggest negative impact on patient satisfaction with the way CGH manages DRG 127, and it suggests that patients experience problems while being treated and do not particularly like the way the problem is resolved—if it is resolved at all. But what problems are we talking about? The item that is a close second for priority reflects empowerment. Would patients continue to feel that their problems went unresolved if they had more participation in their own medical management?

By focusing on the surveys of DRG 127 patients, we could look for the lowest-scoring items and assume that these issues generated problems that went unresolved. We could run correlation coefficients between the service recovery question and all other items on the survey to see which are most highly linked with service recovery. These issues, if low scoring, likely underlie the low score for staff response to problems or concerns. Staff brainstorming, or even a focus group of patients treated for DRG 127, might help CGH arrive at a solution.

Again, I must stress that surveys alone cannot identify the root causes of low satisfaction scores. Once you have identified the existence of a problem, identifying the underlying cause and an effective solution are up to you.

CONCLUSIONS

The deeper you dig into satisfaction data, the more insights you can derive. Through a series of demographic questions on the survey itself, you can generate basic data on patient age, sex, payer, length of stay, and so forth. When you run these against patient satisfaction, you can get closer to identifying the root causes of problems. This saves time, money, and personnel and lets you be more effective in your improvement programs.

To analyze patient satisfaction data by physician, DRG, major diagnostic category (MDC), usage, and costs, you will need to include an identifier on the survey so you can access data derived from specific cases. Of course, you will analyze and report these analyses in the aggregate, not by individual patient. By knowing what patients think of services that generate your greatest volume and profit, you can protect your bottom line and market share and improve care for the maximum number of patients.

Of course, your core mission is to provide care for sick people, not to make money, but if you cannot sustain market share or keep out of the red, then you will not be around to provide care, regardless of how high its quality. Thus, being able to link profit and patient satisfaction to specific conditions or procedures provides important insights for priority setting. Do not apologize for selecting QI targets based on volume. Improving the quality of care for any condition is justified and laudable—especially if your efforts affect a larger number of patients.

ACTION FOR SATISFACTION

1. Include a patient identifier—possibly a barcode or number—on each survey.
2. Ask a number of demographic questions on age, sex, and so forth if you cannot use an identifier so you can do some quick, easy, in-depth analyses without having to go to archived records for these data. However, be careful not to stray into market research territory. Avoid questions that solicit income or other kinds of information that suggest the survey is less for quality improvement than sales improvement.
3. Examine low-scoring items by the demographic data. This helps zero in on causes of problems. Say, for example, that patients who rate you lowest for a particular issue are women between the ages of 30 and 50. This may give you a clue to directions for satisfaction improvement efforts. If you still cannot figure out why these patients are dissatisfied, then at the very least you have a good idea of the most effective composition of a focus group.

4. Analyze satisfaction data by clinical (e.g., DRG) and financial (e.g., profit, costs, usage) data. In addition to the insights previously mentioned, you will be able to quantitatively demonstrate the link between patient satisfaction and bottom line. This helps legitimize the place of patient satisfaction within the core organizational culture. Demonstrating these links can encourage commitment by showing that the payoff for attention to patient satisfaction is hard rather than merely soft.

CHAPTER 8

From Data to Action

AN OLD PROVERB: "You can't fatten the cow by weighing it." If you do not have an effective program for addressing and improving patient satisfaction, then you will not get any benefit or joy from measuring it. You cannot blame the survey for low scores. To that end, this chapter focuses on problem solving and offers five ways to avoid common pitfalls in program implementation.

DON'T SHOOT THE MESSENGER

I recently got a call from a client telling me that they wanted to leave for another satisfaction measurement company. Their scores had been relatively flat for several quarters, and they were becoming discouraged. A committee decided that the patient satisfaction survey was not "sensitive" enough. As an example, they discussed the question that asked how well the patient's pain was controlled. The client said that nurses believed the appropriate way to word this question is how well the pain was "managed." "Managed" was a medically relevant term to nurses. They argued that pain could not be completely avoided for some conditions or procedures. "Managed" suggests a more realistic handling of pain. "Controlled," they noted, suggests full remission of pain, which could be unrealistic.

I decided not to go into all of the reasons why their contention made little sense. I did not say that the clinical implication of the word "manage" is not familiar to patients, while "control" is familiar to all. I did not point out that if pain were not fully relieved, then patients would score that question low regardless of which word was used. On the other hand, if patients were given realistic explanations of expected pain and the limitations of analgesic methods, then the scores would be higher regardless of which word was used.

In short, this hospital's administration believed that satisfaction scores would increase if the questionnaire were worded differently. The questionnaire was to blame for their flat scores. If the questionnaire were different, then the patients would be more satisfied (maybe their pain would even go away!), and the hospital would not have to lift a finger to improve anything.

Of course, I could not say all this. It was a clear case of shooting the messenger. I did not want to confront them about spending more time criticizing the survey than responding to the data.

The point of these examples is clear: Measurement is not management. Satisfaction data provide a starting point only, and then the real work begins. The best data in the world are worthless if not taken seriously or not used. Mary Malone, an independent quality improvement consultant, wryly notes that

Over the past ten years, I've gotten various calls from hospitals demanding an explanation for their satisfaction scores. They say, "Our scores are down, and we don't know why!" At the same time, in all those years not one ever called me to say, "Our scores are *up*, and we don't know why!" Frankly, they're not calling us because they know why their scores are up. Up or down, they don't know why because they never investigate. When they're doing well, they take it for granted. They don't attempt to find out what they're doing right so they can duplicate it in problem areas or if their scores start to take a dip. When they're doing poorly, they call us rather than turn inward to identify and address problems.

GO BEYOND THE NUMBERS FOR INSIGHT

Survey data are limited by the number and specificity of questions that are asked. Insight is also limited by the number of demographic and other pieces of data you collect from patients. Combining your survey data with other patient data may tell you that younger female patients with a particular DRG and shorter length of stay are more dissatisfied than others. But this still does not pinpoint the effective cause of dissatisfaction.

The bottom line is this: When you have finally wrung all the data dry, dug into the numbers, and mulled over the comments, the solution to the problem rests with you, not the survey.

Brainstorming when the Patient "Gets it Wrong"

To the patient, perception is reality. Let's say that patients are giving you low scores for how well their pain was controlled. You have reviewed your procedures and have come to the conclusion that nurses are indeed following state-of-the-art protocols for pain management. Is the patient simply wrong? Maybe, but that is irrelevant. Regardless of what is really happening, patients will still tell others that your staff do not care enough about patient comfort.

With the data in, it is time to brainstorm. Discussions with staff may suggest that what is really going on is that patients are not informed sufficiently about the kind of pain that is common with their condition and the limitations of medications for that pain. Thus, their expectations are unrealistic. You cannot get this insight directly from a single pain-control question on the survey. Of course, you could ask several additional pain-related questions, but there is no guarantee that patients' perception of pain management will be limited to these issues. Certainly, patients will not be able to judge behind-the-scenes decisions or practices that result in perceptions of insufficient pain control.

One hospital was getting frequent negative comments and low scores for daily cleaning of rooms. At the same time, housekeeping staff insisted that the rooms were adequately cleaned. They distrusted the survey data and complained about the numbers. They felt that either the patients or the data were wrong.

The survey manager at the hospital sliced and diced the data, but the only potentially meaningful pattern that emerged was an indication that the bulk of low scores and negative comments came from several units in the hospital's older wing.

It was time to go beyond the data. A discussion group was formed that included nursing and housekeeping staff from the low-scoring units, plus a few housekeeping staff from other units. Then, a tour of the target units was organized. Back around the table, the group dismissed the possibility that patients were judging the rooms to be dirty because they were older. Although the wing was indeed older, it had been recently refurbished and had bright colors, cheerful decor, good floor coverings, windows, and so forth. The rooms did not look or feel old. It was also found that staff who cleaned these units also cleaned other hospital units that had high scores for cleaning. So, it did not appear to be a staff competence issue.

One thing about the units did stand out, however: The rooms were organized in pairs. Two private rooms shared a common bath. In discussing the procedures that were typically used, it was discovered that housekeeping personnel entered one room, cleaned it, went into the bathroom and cleaned that, and then entered the adjoining room from the bathroom and cleaned it, finally departing through the corridor door of the second room.

A lengthy discussion suggested that two things might be happening: (1) when staff departed the first room via the bath, the patient perceived no clear closure of the act of cleaning; and (2) by entering the second room via the bath, the cleaning person somewhat compromised the second patient's privacy. This brainstorming led to a simple solution. After cleaning the first room and bath, the housekeeping staff member exited that same room and was scripted to say, "There, your room is clean. Is there anything more I can do for you?" This clearly informed the patient that the cleaning had been done (closure). By entering the second room through the corridor door, the perception of privacy-intrusion was eliminated. Housekeeping scores rose, and negative comments declined.

An Exercise in Problem Solving

You have low scores for promptness of nurse response to the call button. You drill down into the survey data to see if the problem is ongoing or seasonal, gender or age related, and widespread or limited to a few nursing units. After you have exhausted insights from the data, bring your own insights to the table.

Constructing a "fishbone" chart is useful in organizing a search for causes of a low-scoring issue. The design of the chart is important, as the organizing categories you choose (the major "bones") will invariably direct your thinking to causes that fit the categories.

Regardless of the specific issue to be tackled, your fishbone chart should begin with two major categories or divisions: hospital causes and patient causes. Hospital causes are under the control of the institution. Patient causes refer to characteristics of patients that could affect their perception of care. Subcategories should reflect major logical elements. Hospital causes can be broken into three major subcategories: organization, environment, and personnel. Patient causes can be broken into three causal categories: condition, culture, and personality.

Hospital *organization* refers to roles, rules, rituals, job descriptions, and processes by which staff get things done. *Environment* refers to the ways in which the physical plant (e.g., rooms, layout, construction, ambiance), machinery, and objects affect what gets done. *Personnel* refers to staff personal values and characteristics resulting from race, ethnicity, social class, professional identity, past experiences, and personality.

Patient *condition* refers to both the specific medical problem, the treatment and prognosis of which could produce varying degrees of anxiety, and the physical condition, which itself can produce discomfort and disability as well as resulting anxiety. *Culture* refers to the beliefs, practices, and expectations about health, treatment, and patienthood that the patient brings to the hospital. Ethnic group identity can play a large role here. As indicated in Chapter 5, these beliefs and expectations can clash with standard clinical values and practices. *Personality* refers to idiosyncratic personal characteristics brought to the hospital. These characteristics can result from patient age, sex, professional or domestic identity, past experiences, and so forth.

In any instance where patients give you a low score, assume that the cause can lie either with you or the patient, or both. With the major bones of the chart identified, you can more easily identify specific situations or behaviors that can cause the problem.

The cause-and-effect fishbone diagram in Figure 8.1 does not identify all possible causes, nor are all the categories listed relevant to your institution. You will be able to add a number of other categories.

Patient causes have an effect on patient perceptions that nurses are not responding quickly enough to the call button. These perceptions may or may not be realistic. Hospital causes reflect genuine delays in response that are ostensibly within the control of the institution. Often, delays may not be substantial but are viewed as such by anxious patients. Thus, delays are both real and perceptual at the same time. The solution would involve both interactions with the patient plus organizational, procedural, or mechanical changes by the hospital.

For each possible cause, develop several possible solutions. For example, hospital environmental causes may involve a broken call button. Check daily to see if they are all in working order. Does the call signal outside the door or at the nursing station sometimes fail? Can nurses see or hear the signal if away from the station? Is the call button easily found by the patient? Is it part of the television

Figure 8.1. Cause-and-Effect Fishbone Diagram

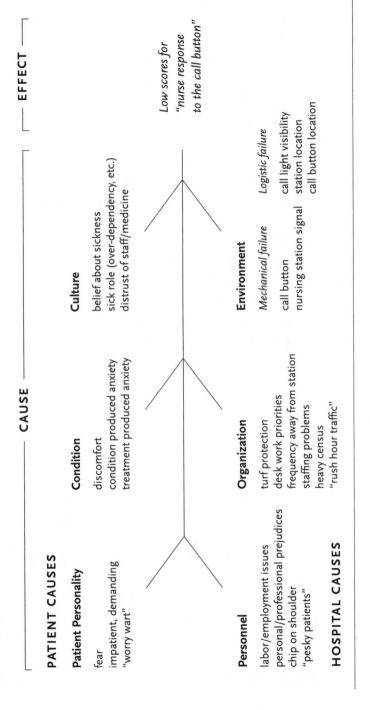

CAUSE — EFFECT

PATIENT CAUSES

Patient Personality

fear
impatient, demanding
"worry wart"

Condition

discomfort
condition produced anxiety
treatment produced anxiety

Culture

belief about sickness
sick role (over-dependency, etc.)
distrust of staff/medicine

*Low scores for
"nurse response
to the call button"*

Personnel

labor/employment issues
personal/professional prejudices
chip on shoulder
"pesky patients"

Organization

turf protection
desk work priorities
frequency away from station
staffing problems
heavy census
"rush hour traffic"

Environment

Mechanical failure

call button
nursing station signal

Logistic failure

call light visibility
station location
call button location

HOSPITAL CAUSES

control pad (thus being one button among many—patients are often confused by this)? Perhaps nurses should test patients' knowledge an hour or two after admission by asking them to identify and press the call button. They may have forgotten or become confused during the initial flurry of instructions and settling in.

Invariably, you will view some hospital causes as beyond your control. For example, paperwork at the nursing station is continual and mandatory, consuming time that nurses could otherwise spend with patients. Unanticipated staffing shortages or an unusually high census cannot be controlled. Nurses are frequently called away from the station for very legitimate reasons and may not see or hear the call signal.

Are these delay-producing situations thus beyond reach? Not if you want to modify their negative effect on patients! Nurses could carry call beepers. Protocols could be developed that allow any hospital employee in the vicinity, not just nurses, to answer a call button. A situationally high census could result in the hiring of additional agency nurses if the hospital is willing to hit the budget for the expense. Remember that all work rules and protocols are culture—a product of decisions and rituals—and thus subject to modification.

Using Comments that Patients Write on Surveys

Comments written by patients are essentially the simplest, most direct and universally comprehensible pieces of data on the survey. Comments can be invaluable. Usually, they are short and general (e.g., "Nurses were great!"). Often enough, however, they are specific and go into some detail about a good or bad experience with named procedures, individuals, or types of staff.

Written comments by patients help you identify specific problems as well as processes that are working especially well. Each department and unit should receive copies of all comments, both positive and negative. Posting surveys bearing positive comments in a place where both staff and patients can see them serves to reinforce the culture. Schedule periodic sessions in which staff discuss the negative comments and attempt to identify underlying causes.

Few comments on returned surveys actually name specific staff members. If a specific staff member is named in a negative comment, then it is not necessary to confront the issue unless it appears to be a pattern. If several different patients make the same complaint, the staff member's supervisor should discuss the issue with him or her.

Positive comments that identify an employee by name should always be sent to the top executive officer, who in turn should send a brief congratulatory note to the employee. At most, a couple of these might arrive each day; writing such notes will not compromise an executive's time. If Judy, a nurse on 3W, receives a copy of the survey bearing the positive comment with a congratulatory scribble from the CEO, this is powerful reinforcement indeed—and it costs nothing.

You can use a word processing program with your survey comments to seek out keywords (e.g., procedures, physicians, nurses, units, services) that help you identify targets for reward or improvement.

SET GOALS FOR PATIENT SATISFACTION

When you have identified the possible cause underlying a problem, you will then develop a plan of action for improvement. To monitor your plan, you will need to establish goals. This is especially necessary if staff performance evaluation and/or compensation are based to some extent on patient satisfaction scores. Some issues that concern goal setting are as follows:

1. *Never set satisfaction score goals without first establishing a plan of action that should have an effect on the scores*; otherwise, expect frustration and disillusionment.

2. *Make the timetable realistic.* Make sure you establish a realistic timetable for realizing your goals. Several measurement periods may be required to implement changes and give them a chance to begin having a full impact on patients. If you note a low-scoring item in your latest quarterly data report and subsequently implement problem solving and QI activities, then you have to give the team time to get up to speed. Do not expect to see an improvement in scores three short months later. Sometimes, longer-term goals are appropriate. Short-term goals are useful only where obvious quick fixes are possible and where there is enough time for the fix to be picked up by the survey.

3. *Make the goal itself realistic.* Regardless of the method and the timetable, the goal itself must be realistic. It is easy enough to say, "We want to be the best in the country," but achieving it may be all but impossible. Whether your overall satisfaction score is based on a single question or is derived from the scores of all the individual questions on the survey, you will have to address dozens of subsidiary issues to improve the overall score. Thus, improvement in overall score is harder to achieve. Improvements in individual survey items are easier and quicker to attain. Setting overall improvement goals of half a point to a full point is realistic. For specific, individual issues, setting improvement goals of two or three points is realistic.

It is also unrealistic to expect all aspects of the patient's hospital experience to provide 100 percent satisfaction. You will never get food scores to equal nursing scores (if you do, then there is something very wrong with your nursing!). You cannot legitimately compare lab with nursing, or physicians with admitting. Patients encounter each of these with different expectations and evaluate each on a different basis. Keep departmental evaluations separate. Pit food service satisfaction scores against peer-group food scores or your own past food scores, not against present nursing scores.

4. *Do not go for the Big Kahuna.* Again, use external information cautiously. Do not focus on the highest score achieved nationally and adopt it as your own goal. Hospital culture, size, location, community, patient constituency, and many other factors affect patient satisfaction. For example, there is a difference of three to five points in overall satisfaction scores between the smallest and largest hospitals. The same goes for hospitals in small towns versus large urban centers. Setting extremely aggressive goals by attempting to match scores of institutions with different demographic characteristics might lead to frustration and reduced commitment on the part of your staff.

A good way to use peer achievements as a goal is to focus on improvement per se rather than on achieving a particular score. If you have an external provider, then ask them to identify the score improvements over the past year of, say, five peer hospitals that match yours in demographic characteristics. The hospitals need not be identified. Some of them might even be relatively low scoring but have improved significantly. Use the average improvement achieved by those five hospitals as your own goal. If they can improve scores for the information patients were given about caring for oneself at home after discharge by three points, then you can do it, too!

Set realistic goals that are achievable. Focus on a limited number of issues at a time. The more specific these issues are, the more chance of success. Remember that your goals may change with time. At first, goals will likely be internally guided. In a second phase, you might want to focus on issues that have an effect on your positioning among peers. In a final phase, after you have improved and your satisfaction scores are beginning to level off, focus on maintaining rather than improving your performance; this may involve tweaking rather than significant intervention. Hospitals near the top in performance may have difficulty sustaining the excitement and commitment that drove earlier phases of the improvement plan. Constant reaffirmation may be needed. Bold improvement plans are far less important than motivational programs.

5. *Set interim goals.* Establish a series of smaller goals rather than aim strictly for the top. Interim goals have the advantage of being more readily achievable and give staff some continual reinforcement along the way to the top. Thunderbird Samaritan Medical Center in Glendale, Arizona, threw a 1950s-themed party when they hit the 50th percentile in their peer group, a '60s party when they hit the 60th, and, subsequently, a '70s event where the CEO donned an Elvis costume. This is strong reinforcement that keeps goals—and their achievement—continually fresh.

6. *Establish internal goals.* You can base goals on either internal or external referents. Internal referents are your own institution's previous satisfaction scores. Goals are set by establishing target increases for the next measurement period. You can pick an arbitrary target number or one that represents a particular percentage increase over the previous score.

   Keep in mind that the range of scores is typically narrow. Within any given hospital, for example, a ten-point difference might be all that separates the highest and lowest scoring nursing units. Do not pick an unrealistically large jump as your goal. If you have a nursing score of 82, then setting a goal of a 10 percent increase means a whopping (and unrealistic) eight-point jump. If your usual spread of nursing scores is, say, ten points, then eight points would actually constitute an 80 percent increase! With a ten-point spread, a more realistic goal of 10 percent would be only a single point.

7. *Pick a statistically significant increase.* Pick a number that represents a statistically significant increase over the previous score. In this case, t-tests are used to identify target numbers that represent confidence levels of .1, .05, .01, and so forth. Hitting these targets indicates that your numbers are 90, 95,

or 99 percent likely to be real rather than a result of chance fluctuation.

If you are measuring satisfaction quarterly, then your score from one quarter to the next may go up in increments too small to reflect statistical significance. At the same time, the increase over a full year may become significant.

As a general rule of thumb, the more surveys you get back, the tighter your confidence intervals—meaning a smaller increase will be statistically significant. If you are working with 200 returned surveys, then an increase or decrease in score of two or three points from the previous period may not be statistically significant. With 400 or 600 returned surveys, however, a variation of but one point might indicate you had achieved your goal—or identified a problem. Remember that we are talking about the actual number of surveys returned (the "n"), not the percentage of the sampled patients who return the survey (the return rate).

8. *Focus on reducing dissatisfiers.* You can also set goals based on something other than mean scores. For example, your patient satisfaction survey probably uses a five-point scale (e.g., "very good" to "very poor," "excellent" to "poor"). If you have a "very good—good—fair—poor—very poor" answer scale, then monitor the number of "poors" and/or "very poors" each quarter and set a goal of reducing them by, say, 5 or 10 percent.

9. *Quantify written comments for goal setting.* Quantify the comments that patients write on their returned surveys by simply counting the number of positive and negative comments. This can be done for the whole hospital or for individual questions, departments, or units. If the ratio of positives to negatives is, say, 4.3 to 1, then set a goal of improving the ratio by 10 percent (4.7 to 1).

10. *Establish externally based goals.* Establish goals by attempting to achieve a particular ranking among your peers. For this, subscribe to an external satisfaction measurement service that

can provide you with access to its national database. The satisfaction scores for most hospitals, as with any frequency distribution, cluster around a national mean. As mentioned above, this mean tends to be fairly high and the range of scores fairly narrow.

Thus, if you are one of the many hospitals clustering between, say, the 40th and 60th percentiles, then a tenth of a point up or down in your mean score could move you up or down quite a few percentage points in the database (this depends, of course, on how large the database is). Toward the upper and lower ends of the national distribution, scores tend to spread out more. This means that you will need more improvement to move from the 80th to the 90th percentile than from the 40th to the 50th percentile. Obtain from your satisfaction measurement provider a printout that shows the mean score associated with each percentile position within its national database. This will allow you to set a percentile-rank goal that reflects a realistic and achievable improvement in your mean score.

Externally based percentile ranks actually offer a useful and valid way of comparing very different services. Food service scores, as were noted, will always be lower than nursing scores, and the two cannot be legitimately compared. Your food scores may be six or seven points lower than your nursing scores, but if your nursing scores put you in the 22nd percentile nationally (against other hospitals' nursing scores), and your food service scores are in the 80th percentile, then your food service is outperforming your nurses (recall Figure 6.11). Knowing this, set more aggressive goals for nursing and less aggressive ones for your dietary department. Dietary is already doing well.

CONCLUSIONS

If you are using sound, adequate survey methodology and have some low scores, then avoid the temptation to shoot the messenger.

Even if you do trust the results, you still have to do something about them. Measurement is not management. The survey is only a starting point. It identifies but not solves your problems.

Patient satisfaction surveys measure patients' perceptions of care. Patients can be "wrong." They may complain about something that is not actually happening, but the result is the same as if the patients were "right." If the patient perceives response to the call button as being slow, then it is slow. If the room is perceived as dirty, then it is dirty, and that is what the patients will tell their friends and relatives. You measure patient satisfaction to tap patient perceptions—not objective clinical reality. If you wanted to measure what is really going on, then you would not be asking patients. Thus, to improve satisfaction with care, you must address both the care and the patient's perceptions.

When you have designed strategies to address these issues—and only then—you can set goals for patient satisfaction. Make sure the goals are realistic and achievable.

ACTION FOR SATISFACTION

1. Involve all managers and team leaders from the beginning. This ensures that the survey itself will be taken seriously. Well before your first survey is even printed, hold discussions about the questions and what they might mean to patients. A team of nurses should go over the nursing questions, for example. Ask your survey director or outside contractor to explain and defend the rationale for any survey question about which staff may have doubts. When staff have signed off on the survey, they cannot easily complain later that it is not appropriate.
2. Practice problem solving well before the first survey results are in. Nurses should address each nursing item on the survey, attempting to identify causes that could underlie a low score. Be methodical in these brainstorming sessions. Have staff practice creating cause-effect or fishbone diagrams for selected items

on the survey. With major discussion categories preselected (i.e., patient causes versus hospital causes and their major subcategories), staff will be less likely to focus on peripheral (or less personally threatening) explanations rather than more subtle, in-depth possible causes of low scores.

3. Make survey score goals achievable. Set a series of smaller, shorter-term, easily reached goals rather than requiring a single big leap that takes a longer period of time to achieve. Short-term achievable goals reinforce commitment by offering regular rewards. Go for half a point improvement over six months rather than a full point over a year.

CHAPTER 9

From Action to Satisfaction—
Creating a Culture,
Not Just a Program

ALL SOCIAL BEHAVIOR occurs within a cultural context. Each cultural context facilitates particular behaviors and discourages others. To affect lasting change in your institution, you have to change the culture. I like the motto created by Memorial Hospital Pembroke in Pembroke Pines, Florida, for their patient satisfaction effort: "It's not a program—it's a culture!" Holy Cross Hospital in Chicago, Illinois, explained their high scores: "Our mission isn't just hanging framed on the wall."

There is such a thing as a patient satisfaction culture. It consists of organizational values, beliefs, roles, and behaviors that encourage a special connection between caregivers and patients. This special connection facilitates the flow of empathy and information between patients and all caregivers in the organization. Like any culture, its members must believe in it for it to work. "Believe in" means that the culture is taken for granted and requires no special motivation or reward. Patient satisfaction becomes automatic, and it is simply "the thing to do." Mayer and Cates (2004, xix) are adamant in stating that "all fundamental, meaningful, and lasting change is intrinsically rather than extrinsically motivated."

You cannot mandate concern for patient satisfaction if staff think it is merely fluff. You cannot demand that staff take patient satisfaction seriously if they do not feel they will be rewarded for trying. You cannot mandate it if they perceive that the task is theirs but not an equal concern of top management. You cannot have significant improvement if patient satisfaction is not tied directly to the job evaluation of every person in the organization, from top to bottom. If your department heads and top managers do not know your latest patient satisfaction scores, then you are not yet poised for significant improvement. If patient satisfaction is not a permanent agenda item at all meetings of all groups, including the board of trustees and medical staff, then the satisfaction-facilitating cultural context is not present.

You are also not ready to make a significant impact on your patients' satisfaction if you think your hospital is different from others. It isn't!

Remember that the patient—not you—experiences, perceives, and evaluates care. Whether your facility is old or new, in an upper class neighborhood or inner city, a large teaching hospital in a big city or a rural institution with but a single nursing unit—all patients want the same thing from you. They want relevant, intelligible explanations about what is being done. They want competent technical care. They want prompt response to the call button. They want respect, friendliness, and empathy from nurses and all other staff with whom they come in contact. They want appropriate pain control. They want promises kept. They want tasty meals and a cheerful room. They want this and a lot more from every hospital, ED, or clinic in the country. Whether your patients are predominantly sicker, older, younger, richer, or less affluent than the average does not matter. No excuse is valid for slow response to the call button, poor pain management, cursory explanations, or apparent lack of empathy for the personal effects of the sickness.

I am not saying that patients at all hospitals are alike. Your patients in general probably do indeed differ from patients at other hospitals with different customer demographics—but the point is that this does not matter. Your job is to thoroughly familiarize yourself with your particular patient constituency and shape your approach to care so that their satisfaction is maximized. If you automatically adjust your medical treatment (e.g., dosages) to accommodate a patient's diagnosis, age, weight, physical condition, and so forth, then why would it not be appropriate to adjust behavioral and interactive protocols to fit patient needs that might derive from their condition, age, sex, social class, education level, ethnicity, or other demographic characteristics? You must learn who your patients are and what they want from you.

You cannot blame your patients for lower satisfaction scores. Blame justifies inaction.

WHAT DO WE MEAN BY "CULTURE"?

Concern for patient satisfaction operates within a cultural context that facilitates it. Culture is not a simple concept. Culture is a complex bag that governs meanings, values, attitudes, and behaviors for a particular group of people.

A hospital's culture thus involves far more than a mission statement or official published policies. Staff attitudes toward each other, patients, and administration are culture. When staff say, "We always do X this way," or "We don't have the money to remodel the ED," or "Medicaid patients push the call button too much," or "Administration doesn't care about the stress we're under," or "Only nurses should pass food trays because nurses know what patients should or shouldn't be eating," they are talking about culture. Formal (idealized) job descriptions are culture. At the same time, the way in which jobs are really perceived and carried out is culture. The prejudices and attitudes (e.g., professional, racial, economic, ethnic, political, religious) brought to the hospital by staff are culture. The ways in which these prejudices and attitudes are tolerated, facilitated—or minimized—in the hospital setting are culture.

Here is an example of culture at work.

Jake, one of our account executives, reported that he recently visited two hospitals located in the same town. It was raining heavily when he got to the first hospital's parking lot. As he contemplated getting out of his car in the downpour, a covered golf cart pulled up alongside him. He was given a dry lift to the hospital entrance.

Once inside, he approached the reception desk. He asked if the clerk could phone a particular department head and tell her he was here for his appointment. "Sure thing," said the clerk. "If you wait here a minute, I'll get someone to take you there." The clerk looked the number up, made the call, and got someone to take Jake upstairs.

Jake's visit to the second hospital a couple of hours later was quite different. It was still pouring. This time, there was no golf cart in the parking lot to give him a lift. Soaking, he ran to the canopied entrance only to find a covered golf cart sitting there with the driver lounging on the seat. "Why aren't you out there fetching people?" asked Jake.

"It's raining," explained the driver.

Once inside, he approached the reception desk and asked the clerk if she'd contact a particular department head.

"Do you have their phone number?" asked the clerk.

"No," answered Jake. "Could you please look it up for me?"

The clerk balked at this, stating that she had a lot of papers to go through to find the number. Jake said never mind and searched through his briefcase until he came across the number. He gave it to the clerk, who attempted to call. There was no answer.

Jake said he'd just go on up. Could the clerk give him directions?

"Well, it's rather difficult," replied the clerk. "You go down that corridor there until . . ." The directions were complex, and Jake had to ask another person along the way.

These hospitals have two very different corporate cultures. Guess which hospital has higher patient satisfaction scores?

Cultures Are Learned

Cultures are passed from one generation or group of staff to the next through both informal and formal interaction. Each hospital has a unique culture, and this culture is learned by new employees. Employees learn the culture primarily by observing and participating in it and mimicking the other staff with whom they work. This is the real, "on the ground," everyday culture. The official culture is of far less importance. It is picked up largely through formal training and may be minimally reflected in actual daily behavior. Formal training in the absence of a satisfaction-facilitating culture will not work.

Culture Is Integrated

An integrated culture means that its parts are typically linked to one another. Actions (e.g., behaviors, expressed attitudes) in one part affect actions in others. This concept is a no-brainer. You will recall that a key element of total quality management is the interdependency of all within the organization. Everyone is simultaneously a receiver of service from some and a provider of service to others. Nurses depend on physicians, pharmacists, and delivery personnel to get meds. Patients depend on nurses for getting the right meds in a timely manner. *Everyone is a middleman in the hospital.* That is why the attitudes and approaches of one department, unit, or specialty affect others up and down the line.

Culture Is Patterned

A patterned culture means that concepts and values expressed in one part of the culture are expressed in other parts as well. For example, if you provide exceptional service in the parking lot and admitting desk, then you are likely giving good information to patients about their treatment. No set of behaviors within the hospital is really insulated from others. What nurses say and do on 4W is heard and observed by lab staff, transporters, admitting clerks, physicians, volunteers, administrators, and every other person who comes in contact with that unit.

By definition, cultures are hard to change. That is because culture is internalized, taken for granted, and expressed institutionwide. Changes introduced in one sector alone could be thwarted by the existing culture in other parts of the institution. In short, cultural change is hard to do piecemeal. Nor can you expect a successful cultural change for line staff if top managers do not share the same set of expectations and values (see Sherman 1997 for an illuminating analysis of organizational changes needed to attain a new level of hospital quality).

All of this means that success is best achieved by attempting to make cultural changes simultaneously institutionwide rather than by testing the waters and focusing piecemeal on individual departments or staff. If culture is not shared and valued by all, then it will not work. And culture cannot be mandated. Cultures, like organisms, evolve. If you can get people performing the proper behavior, then they will likely wind up believing that it is the proper thing to do. Ultimately, they will do it without thinking about it. When a behavior begins to be taken for granted, it is becoming a core part of the culture.

CULTURAL CHARACTERISTICS OF TOP PATIENT SATISFACTION ORGANIZATIONS

The following were distilled from characteristics of award-winning hospitals that partner with Press Ganey Associates in the measurement and improvement of patient satisfaction. Some have achieved "Comeback of the Year" status from *Hospitals and Health Networks*. Others have won national awards, including "Success Story" recognition from Press Ganey for exemplary improvement of patient satisfaction.

Commitment Starts at the Top

In top organizations, the CEO lives the patient satisfaction mission and demands this orientation from everyone else. The CEO knows the hospital's latest survey scores, including the identity of the highest and lowest ranking departments and nursing units. Patient satisfaction issues top meeting agendas and occupy a permanent place on the board of trustees' meeting agenda. The CEO is held accountable for the institution's scores. A significant part of senior management performance evaluations rely on their success with patient satisfaction goals for their departments or areas. The CEO reinforces the orientation by sending a personal note to every employee complimented by patients in letters or surveys. The CEO provides the resources needed to enhance satisfaction. In a financial crunch, patient satisfaction programs are among the last to have their budgets cut.

The Organization Enthusiastically Admits that Patients Are Also Customers

No conflict exists in these organizations over this question. Everyone from valet to chief of medicine buys into the importance of care as customer service and of customer service as care. Combining both top-level commitment and the conviction that patients are customers, Covenant Health System in Lubbock, Texas, introduces staff to their patient satisfaction program with a clear letter from the CEO (see Appendix 9.1).

Satisfaction Programs and Successes Are Publicized Throughout the Institution and Beyond

If patient satisfaction activities go on behind closed doors, they will not enter the culture. Successful hospitals involve all staff through activity and publicity. Many hospitals post all satisfaction scores where everyone can see them. Positive letters and satisfaction surveys with accolades for staff may be pasted on walls throughout the institution for both patients and staff to see. On the one hand, such publicity provides good public relations and tells patients that you really care about what they say; on the other hand, public posting of positive surveys rewards staff and further reinforces the overall importance given to patient satisfaction. Awards and recognition should be continual throughout the year—such repetitive rituals serve to reinforce the culture.

Institutionwide celebrations for improvements in overall satisfaction scores are essential. After all, everyone contributes to the patient's total experience of care. Van Wert County Hospital in Van Wert, Ohio, gave celebratory t-shirts to all staff when they first hit the 99th percentile in patient satisfaction nationally. The next year, when they had sustained their high-scoring position, a hospitalwide pizza party marked the occasion. Van Wert also produced several public-relations commercials on local TV stations, proudly proclaiming their achievements in patient satisfaction.

You probably already have an in-house newsletter. Make sure that patient satisfaction stories and programs are high profile. Two hospital newsletter examples from Bristol Hospital in Bristol, Connecticut, and Columbus Regional Hospital in Columbus, Indiana, include patient satisfaction stories on the front page (see Appendixes 9.2 and 9.3).

Service Recovery Is Viewed as a Key Program Element

Of course, you want to satisfy your patients. But perfection is impossible. It is now gospel in the quality improvement movement that patients experiencing a service failure —and subsequent service repair and/or apology—are actually more satisfied with the hospital than patients who experience and express no problem at all. Indeed, service recovery (e.g., "Staff response to concerns or complaints you may have had during your stay") is one of the issues most highly correlated with the likelihood of patient's recommending the hospital to others (from Press Ganey database of over 2 million patients in 2005). Thus, far from being at best a neutral response to problems, *good complaint management is itself a strong satisfier.*

The basics of an effective program include

1. a clear list of steps to be taken when a patient complains;
2. a concept of ownership of a complaint until it is resolved or another person takes over;
3. protocols for distinguishing between problems that can be addressed by the first person to whom the patient complains versus those issues that should be bumped-up to a higher level;
4. protocols for addressing the complaint verbally;
5. protocols for addressing the complaint behaviorally;
6. protocols for determining when—and to what extent—a patient or family should be compensated (e.g., cash, gift) for the inconvenience or discomfort; and
7. a training program for all of the above, including clear empowerment of staff to handle most service issues without having to first justify a decision to superiors.

Most hospitals have some form of service recovery program. While the acronyms differ, their content is similar. The acronym is useful in that it formalizes the process and the steps to be taken:

Lexington Medical Center (West Columbia, South Carolina)
"GIFT" program
  G = Give a sincere apology
  I = Inform the patient
  F = Fix the problem
  T = Thank the person

Russell Medical Center (Alexander City, Alabama)
"CARE" program

C = Connect with the customer
A = Apologize
R = Respond to the problem
E = Evaluate

St. Luke's Hospital (Bethlehem, Pennsylvania)
"ERASE" program
E = Evaluate the situation
R = Regrets expressed
A = Act immediately
S = Satisfy needs
E = Evaluate

In all of these programs, front line staff have a simple, scripted response to issues raised by patients. Wording can vary (e.g., "I'm sorry that happened," "I'm sorry you've been upset"), but the apology is essential. No blame is acknowledged.

Typically, the staff member who discovers the problem owns it until it is turfed or solved. Even if it is turfed, the person to whom the patient complained still apologizes for the issue. Complaints that should be turned over to supervisors or patient representatives would generally involve medical/treatment issues. These might include medical errors, procedure-generated discomfort such as complaints after multiple attempts to insert an IV, significant information failures, or loss of valued or valuable personal items.

Most complaints are not medical. They typically involve issues such as amenities or personal comfort, noise, meals, communication, interactions with family, and in particular actual or perceived delays. These are issues that can be addressed by all front line staff.

Gifts or compensation should not be offered until the complaint has been resolved.

Resolution means that (1) the issue is fixed and an apology has been given, or (2) the issue cannot be fixed (e.g., the meal is late and you cannot make time run backward) and an apology given. In most instances, a sincere apology brings closure to the issue.

Owning-up to a service failure and making the patient believe that you truly feel bad about it is typically all the patient wants. Thus, wholesale gifting for service failures is usually unnecessary.

Gifting, however, has a dual function of making both patient and staff member feel better about the issue. From this perspective, it may often be unnecessary, yet it serves a good purpose. Gifting usually takes the form of certificates good for various hospital commercial services such as the lunchroom, parking, gift shop, or vending machines. Some programs include flowers or fruit baskets to be given for serious problems. These more expensive gifts are typically made (or at least approved) by supervisors rather than line staff.

Froedtert Hospital in Milwaukee, Wisconsin, has developed a succinct service recovery protocol that includes appropriate stages, actions, scripts, and rationales. As with all successful programs, Froedtert emphasizes that gifts or compensation (e.g., their "All Out Recovery" certificates) are to be given only after all other phases of recovery are complete. Their "All Out Recovery" gift certificates include modest vouchers for the gift shop, cafeteria, and a variety of other services. *Any* staff can distribute these without permission from supervisors. Froedtert estimates the annual cost of such gifting to be around $40,000—a very cheap investment for the good will generated.

The following is a summary of Froedtert's service recovery program:

Service Standard

I recognize customer complaints and concerns are a chance to make things right and serve as opportunities for improvement. I work to resolve them quickly and help create an environment that makes it easy for customers to express concerns.

Protocols

■ I implement "All Out Recovery" following the L.A.S.T. process: Listen, Apologize, Solve, Thank, if a customer complains or is disappointed.

- I actively listen to the customer, without becoming defensive, without interrupting, blaming others or making excuses.
  - **Listen to Understand**—We often listen with the intent to respond, not with the intent to understand. People need to vent when they're upset. Don't interrupt!
- I apologize to the customer because he/she is disappointed.
  - **Apologize**—Apologizing doesn't mean you're admitting you did anything wrong. You're apologizing on behalf of the organization. It's a very important step.
  - **Useful phrases**:
    - *"I'm sorry this happened."*
    - *"I'm sorry that you've had this experience."*
    - *"I'm very sorry. I can see that this has upset you."*
    - *"I'm sorry, that must have been frustrating."*
- I take action to solve the problem. If I can't solve it, I find someone who can.
  - **Solve**—Stay calm! Don't argue, make excuses, or blame anyone or any department at this point. The customer wants his/her problem solved.
  - **Sample solving stage statements**:
    - *"According to what you just said, this is what happened . . ."*
    - *"Let me see if I have this straight, what you said was . . ."*
    - *"Yes, I understand. Let me see if I have a clear picture . . ."*
    Once you understand the problem, the focus shifts to resolving the problem. It's time to make it right.
  - **Sample questions at this point would be**:
    - *"What can I do to make this right for you?"*
    - *"What could I do that would make you feel better about this situation?"*
- I communicate to the customer what steps are being taken and when to expect a response.
  - **Key steps to be completed**:
    - Share your plan of action with the customer.
    - Tell them what you'll do, then do it.
    - Tell the customer you did it.

- I thank the customer for bringing the problem to my attention and for his/her patience/understanding.
  - **Thank—Sample statements**:
    - — *"Thanks for calling this to my attention. I'll discuss this with my supervisor so we can make sure it doesn't happen again."*
    - — *"Thank you for your patience in working with me to solve this. I appreciate your bringing this to my attention."*
    - — *"Thank you for sharing this problem with me. We wouldn't want you to leave feeling unhappy about your experience here."*
- I give the customer an All Out Recovery certificate if it is appropriate/necessary.
  - **Do**:
    - —Have them readily available in your area at all times
    - —Use them freely/often, whenever needed
    - —Give them immediately after L.A.S.T.
  - **Don't**:
    - —Give them if you haven't completed L.A.S.T.
    - —Give them if the mistake is so big that the person would feel insulted; instead follow up in another manner, i.e., with Patient Relations
    - —Give them if there has been a clinical/medical error that's been made.
- We also have drink certificates for a free coffee or soda. While these aren't necessarily all out recovery certificates, they can be used for a short delay or any other appropriate use you determine.
- I take customer complaints/incidents that I feel are beyond my control to my supervisor/manager.

A final word about service recovery gifting: Make sure staff do not feel that they will be punished if they distribute gifts. With few exceptions, we are emphatically *not* talking about responses to reportable medical errors. Patient dissatisfiers and complaints are overwhelmingly caused by nonmedical failures—delays, comfort issues, communication or interpersonal glitches, and unmet prom ises and appointments. Because no complex organization functions perfectly, such dissatisfiers are to be expected as a constant.

This means that if you have a gifting option, then departments or units that distribute far fewer than others (given similar patient loads) should be questioned. Are they committed to the program? Departments that give far more gifts than the average should be viewed as service heroes rather than mistake prone. The good will generated is worth far more than the cost of the meals, shop items, or parking. This is especially the case in situations where the staff member co-opts the situation by responding to a service failure that the patient obviously experienced but did *not* complain about. This is an opportunity for wowing the customer.

Patient Satisfaction Data Are Taken Seriously and Each Report Is Eagerly Awaited

Staff in every department and unit know their latest satisfaction scores and what their trends are. Satisfaction survey results are posted around the hospital, and all know each other's performance.

If the survey and its scores and trends are monopolized by some central office and not shared with all staff, then ownership of patient satisfaction cannot be institutionwide.

Each department head is responsible for an action plan to im prove satisfaction, and the plan is reviewed and updated at regular intervals, such as 90 days. Realistic goals are set. A hospital in the 10th percentile for ED waiting time should not set a one-year 90th percentile target. If progress is not reported, then a new action plan must be presented that analyzes the failure to improve and outlines clear steps for improvement. Management does not view "We're working on it" as an acceptable progress report. Staff view lower-than-expected scores as opportunities for improvement, not occa sions for punishment.

Staff Are Hired and Trained for Service-Relevant Qualities as well as Task-Specific Skills

During hiring interviews, applicants are screened for personality types that reflect an openness to innovation and to appreciating the importance of the patient's views of care. Those who exhibit distrust of the legitimacy of the patient's evaluation of care are not hired. Some hospitals require new recruits to sign a pledge that focuses attention on efforts to promote quality and patient satisfaction (see Appendixes 9.4 and 9.5). New hires typically sign such pledges after reviewing the behavioral standards demanded (see Appendixes 9.6, 9.7, and 9.8).

During training, the fact that institutional financial survival depends upon viewing patients as customers is stressed. No beating around the bush by focusing solely on lofty mission statements. You have to stay in business, and staff should know that patient satisfaction is a key to the hospital's survival—and to their own long-term job security.

Staff recognize that *they* are the hospital. Otherwise, it is just a building. Every individual believes this and understands that every individual has an impact on patient satisfaction—if not directly, then indirectly as a supplier of service to someone who does have direct access to the patient. Every person feels responsible for patient satisfaction.

Any patient stay in the hospital involves multiple contacts and interactions with staff. As emphasized earlier, both staff and patients bring their own attitudes, prejudices, and values to the clinical encounter.

In the highly rated patient satisfaction institution, workshops are conducted on the effect of staff interaction, including personal style, upon patients and their families. Self-reflective sessions are led by behavioral specialists, focusing on the impact of staff personal and professional values upon their interaction with patients. Simplified discussions on the illness/disease dichotomy are scheduled to make staff aware of the complex beliefs, expectations, and experiences brought by patients to the hospital setting. (Remember, simply saying, "Be sensitive to patient beliefs and backgrounds" does not tell you what these differences are or how to deal with them.) Staff must realize that patients have agendas, too, and that these consist of far more than desire for smiles, warm blankets, and generic words of comfort—however nicely scripted they are.

Staff training must also involve sensitization to the elements of the hospital culture that can thwart efforts at maximizing care. The systemic nature of processes, problems, and solutions (e.g., cross-cutting departmental interconnections) are stressed. Discussions about turf and job boundaries are necessary, focusing on the disadvantage of turf protection for patients and for the hospital's mission of quality care.

All of these training elements focus on the legitimacy of the patient's perspective and its effect on care, outcome, and subsequent evaluation of the hospital experience. You also need to educate staff to the importance, legitimacy, and utilization of your patient satisfaction survey.

Training sessions for line staff on the patient satisfaction survey are best done by department or specialty. Copies of the survey are distributed, along with an explanation of methodology. Sample excerpts of the data reports are provided so staff can familiarize themselves with the numbers and how to interpret them. Staff brainstorm about possible causes and solutions for low-scoring survey items. This prepares them for the task ahead and helps demystify the process of responding to the survey data.

There is no single training model that all institutions should use. Cunningham and Malone (1999) note that at Thunderbird Samaritan Medical Center in Glendale, Arizona, all employees must participate in eight hours of experiential training, focusing on compassion, integrity, and excellence. Similarly, Columbus Regional Hospital in Columbus, Indiana, requires that employees take ten hours of classes dealing with the organization's standards of service.

Focusing on leaders as well as general employees, Baptist Health Care in Pensacola, Florida, requires all middle and upper management to spend two days (off site) every three months to receive training on hiring, supervision, communication, and other satisfaction-focused topics.

When Memorial Hospital Pembroke in Pembroke Pines, Florida, undertook its "WOW" customer service program, it designed six educational classes that all staff members had to attend. The classes and the topics they covered were as follows:

1. First Impressions
   - A video of "Do's and Don'ts"
   - "You only have one chance to make a first impression"
   - Disney's approach to impressing the customer
   - Why first impressions are lasting
   - Dressing for success
2. Achieving Excellence
   - Successful customer service organizations—What makes them that way?
   - What makes customer service in healthcare different?
   - The benefits of customer service
   - How to get from where we are to where we want to be—and stay there
   - Begin with the end in mind
3. Customer Service Principles
   - Basic rules of customer service
   - Reasons why patients recommend hospitals
   - Five key concepts of customer service
   - The importance of word of mouth
4. Teamwork
   - Building a strong sense of teamwork
   - Working as part of a customer service team
   - Defining the essential skills needed to provide WOW service
   - How to maintain a positive team in the workforce
   - Interdepartmental cooperation

5. Effective Communications
   - Verbal and nonverbal communication
   - Telephone etiquette
   - Active listening skills
   - Demonstrate to customers that what they have to say is important to you
   - Focus on the customer's needs
   - Avoid interrupting when the customer speaks
   - Verify and clarify what the customer is saying
   - Maintain eye contact
   - Ask questions in an organized sequence
6. Resolving Customer Problems
   - Identify reasons for customer problems
   - Why healthcare is a problem-prone business
   - Problems are the nature of our business (patients and families come to us in an already high state of stress; the family's expectation of care is higher than the patient's; and we deal in highly complicated, confusing systems)
   - Expectations of care continue to grow
   - Increased public attention to healthcare (puts us in spotlight)
   - The common problems and how to resolve them
   - The best way to avoid problems
   - What customers want most and get the least

At the completion of the final class, Memorial invited employees to a WOW luncheon. Reflecting the hospital's serious view of the program, it was actually a formal affair with tablecloths, flowers, china, and a fancy menu. The top administrator spoke and attendees were given their WOW pins.

A final word about training: Do not waste the time and money if a major, institutionwide patient satisfaction program is not in the works. Do not expect maximum effectiveness from staff training if the CEO is not visibly and obviously committed to the program.

Seeds sown on sterile ground will not grow. One hospital we know of (not one mentioned above) spent big bucks on customer service training for employees, sending them in groups or individually for all-day training sessions. At the same time, no overall organizational program was in place to which all staff were committed and that top leadership actively promoted. When staff returned to their departments after the day of training, they returned to an unchanged cultural context and group dynamic unconcerned with working together to improve patient satisfaction. Needless to say, the hospital's satisfaction scores continued to be low.

The Responses to Important Patient Experiences are Scripted

The vast majority of events and processes in the clinical setting are routine and standardized—how to inject this, how to do that. At the same time, given the importance of communication and information exchange with patients, there is good reason to ensure consistency in patient/staff interaction. This, after all, is a major focus of the book! Thus, scripting must be well integrated into the successful hospital's organization.

There is still some distrust among hospital staff of scripted interactions. The distrust is unwarranted because hospitals are *already* scripting almost every aspect of care.

Consider what a theater script does. It specifies *everything* that the audience sees and hears. A script carefully stipulates the appearance and placement of every piece of furniture and decoration on the stage so as to create the proper atmosphere, advance the plot, and facilitate the flow of action. Then, not only is every spoken word scripted, but emotional tone and body language is usually prescribed as well.

The hospital is but another stage. There is scenery. Every corridor, sign, wall hanging, and piece of furniture; every window view, bed placement, and element of bathroom decor—all of these have an impact on the patient's perception of the entire experience. This impact is not haphazard. The decor and physical facility were planned. Moreover, almost every aspect of medical intervention and management is strictly specified. The protocols for preparing, inserting, and monitoring IVs are not open to ad-libbing. The timing of most events (e.g., vitals, blood draws, med deliveries, meal services) is very routine and highly predictable.

In other words, the hospital setting and the major actions that occur within it are already scripted. As in a theater, this script communicates something to patients that affects their mood and expectations.

The only aspects of care that are not strictly scripted are the ongoing verbal interactions between staff and patient. These are mediated through highly individual personalities. This does not mean that scripting interactions is impossible but rather that the successful hospital utilizes it judiciously. Staff could and should not have to memorize large numbers of scripted interactions. It makes the interactions less comfortable. It feels and sounds phony. Still, some scripting is essential. Scripts can be of two types: general and specific.

General scripting. You do not have to mandate the specific words that nurses use on entering a patient's room. It is not critical whether the nurse says "Hi" or "Good morning." These can be left to the individual. However, the *general intent* of the interaction, a friendly salutation of some sort, should be stipulated, with the goal of putting the patient at ease and creating a less stressful atmosphere. General scripting is an automatic product of culture—you know when you have to do something.

Specific scripting. Some specifically worded scripts are so useful that they should be mandated. The following are three of the most important:

1. *"Is there something else I can do for you?"* Every physician, nurse, food service, and housekeeping staff member should ask this

prior to leaving the room. Moreover, they must stand still and face the patient as they say this and not drop it casually over their shoulder as they walk out the door. This is not done just to be nice. There are positive reasons for this script. It tells patients that it is okay to ask questions or request additional service.

It is also good for staff. Mary Malone, a patient satisfaction consultant, reports on the advantage of such scripting. In one hospital she worked with, two nursing units were selected for a test of the effectiveness of scripting. All staff on one of the units were required to ask patients, "Is there something else I can do for you" prior to leaving the room.

Call button pushes on that unit subsequently dropped by 40 percent! This saved nurses a lot of time.

2. *"Do you have any questions?"* Every time a patient is given a medication, treatment, test, or instructions, the physician, nurse, or technologist should ask this. Note that the script requires the speaker to either sit next to the patient or, at the very least, ask the question while standing at the bedside, facing the patient, with a hand on the patient or bed. This communicates sincerity and can stimulate trust. When patients ask more questions, there is less likelihood of errors or service gaffs.

3. *"I'm really sorry about that."* Whenever a patient complains about something, the person to whom he or she complains should say something like this. Such a statement covers both sins of omission and commission. It is a confirmation of the patient's dissatisfaction and indicates that he or she is taken seriously rather than defensively. At the same time (as mentioned earlier in this chapter), it implies no responsibility or obligation on the part of the speaker or the hospital. Some things can be resolved on the spot. Others must be turfed. Either way, an immediate indication of regret for the dissatisfaction helps defuse the situation and establishes the hospital as empathetic.

Some hospitals script a discharge salutation, such as "It's been a pleasure taking care of you." This is not a bad idea so long as only *one* staff member—ideally the patient's regular nurse—is designated to say it. If more than one person recites this, then it begins to sound like a line and its impact is weakened.

Specific scripts should be limited to key situations where specific words have proven to be of great value. Over-reliance on multiple scripts to be memorized can place a burden on staff while implying that you have little confidence in their ability to act appropriately. You can employ a far greater number of general intent scripts because they require only a simple recognition of the required *nature* of the interaction in certain situations.

Scripting can be useful in every department or service. CentraState Medical Center in Freehold, New Jersey, noted low scores for physician-related items on the emergency patient survey. The low-scoring issues were essentially interactional. For each issue, a simple script was developed to improve communication. Michael Jones, M.D., chairman of the ED, worked with staff physicians to develop a number of scripted statements. Because the importance of patient satisfaction improvement was stressed and because the effort was led by the ED chief, himself a physician, resistance was minimal. The scripts had the following characteristics:

- Easy to memorize (no need to refer to a written prompter and more likely to encourage physician compliance)
- Reflected the wording of a survey item that was an improvement target
- Reflected empathy or concern on the part of the physician

Scripted behavior or communications were created for the following five survey issues:

1. *Courtesy of the physician.*
   Scripts:
   —"Hello, I'm Dr. _____, and I'm here to take care of you."

—Address the patient formally, not by first name.

—Do not ignore accompanying family.

2. *Degree to which the physician took your problem seriously.*
   Scripts:
   —"I'm sorry this happened to you. We'll take good care of you."
   —"This must have been a very (fill in appropriate word: painful, frightening, upsetting, etc.) experience for you."
   —"I can see that you are . . ."
   —"It sounds like what you're telling me is . . ."
   For this issue, the group scripted simple behaviors as well:
   —Make eye contact.
   —Nod in response, or say "uh huh" to show you are listening.
   —If at all possible, sit. Do not stand next to the patient.

3. *Physician's concern for your comfort while treating you.*
   Scripts:
   —"I see you're in pain. Let me . . . (fill in what you plan to do)"
   —"We want to make you as comfortable as possible."

4. *Physician's concern to explain your tests and treatments.*
   Script: "If there's anything you don't understand, please stop me."

5. *Advice you were given about caring for yourself at home.*
   Scripts:
   —"Here's what you can expect . . ."
   —"Here's what you need to do when you leave here . . . (fill in with clear, written discharge instructions)"

It is really not necessary that specific lines be memorized. Again, if staff buy into the general script for each situation, then they can use their own words.

CentraState's ED scores rose significantly and other specialty areas within the hospital began to develop simple scripts for staff to use in common situations (Gutter and Marinaro 2002).

Staff Are Empowered to Provide Exceptional Service

At a top patient satisfaction organization, staff feel permitted to spend a bit more time with patients when they judge it to be necessary. If a patient expresses a need, then staff can fill it, if it is within their abilities. As Eisenberg (1997, 30) notes, "the less empowered the employees, the greater the delay in satisfying the customer." Empowerment also entails a recognition that turf boundaries can be crossed for the sake of patient satisfaction. For example, a housekeeping staff member can refill a patient's ice water or make a phone call to a relative without feeling that it "isn't in my job description" or "I'm stepping on someone else's territory."

Some hospitals empower all levels of staff to provide at least token restitution (e.g., gift or certificate from the hospital gift shop) when they believe patients have experienced some form of service failure. Employees at Holy Cross Hospital in Chicago, Illinois, are authorized to spend up to $250 per patient for service recovery. Staff tend not to go overboard in this, and the total cost is typically negligible—the very act of empowering employees in this way creates a heightened sense of responsibility for and to the institution.

Service recovery (i.e., how well complaints or problems are handled) is one of the survey items most highly correlated with overall satisfaction with care. Service recovery is facilitated when all staff are empowered to participate.

Staff Reward Each Other for Their Patient Satisfaction Orientation

When staff reward each other for patient satisfaction, it reflects a real buy-in on the part of staff. Do what you can to encourage it. Many variations of this type of program exist, but the theme is pretty consistent. Staff member A, observing staff member B do something special for a patient, awards B a certificate of recognition on the spot. Those who accumulate sufficient accolades from their peers receive a special reward from management (e.g., cash, gift certificate, write-up in the staff newsletter).

Many different names exist for these peer-recognition programs. Albany Medical Center in Albany, New York, has a "Giraffe Award" given by a staff member to another who is judged to have "stuck his or her neck out" for a patient. Another hospital has a "Caught in the Act" award.

At Columbus Regional Hospital in Columbus, Indiana, employees can send a "Care-Gram" to another employee judged to be providing exceptional service to patients. Furthermore, when an employee is mentioned positively on the patient survey, he or she is given two carnations by the CEO. The honored individual then has to give one of the flowers to another employee who, behind the scenes, has contributed to the exceptional service praised on the survey. (This is a great idea because it calls attention to the integrated, interdepartmental, systemic nature of care.)

Clara Maass Medical Center in Belleville, New Jersey, implemented a "Just Desserts" program in which complimentary dessert certificates, redeemable at the hospital cafeteria, are periodically handed out to both patients and staff for presentation to employees judged to render exemplary customer service.

Baptist Health Care in Pensacola, Florida, developed a WOW program that concentrates on looking for employees who provide outstanding customer service. Staff who are "caught" by their own or any other manager or administrator are recognized on the spot with a hot pink WOW card. Employees who receive five WOW cards are given a $15 gift certificate to a local business by their manager. Certificate winners' names and the number of WOW cards they have been awarded are published monthly in the newsletter. When the program began, Baptist instituted few rules and no limits to the number of awards an employee could receive. Some staff, of course, were consistent WOW winners because of their special commitment to core issues of patient satisfaction. Baptist did not worry about some individuals monopolizing the awards, because the behavior of these consistent winners could serve as a model for others.

Many hospitals have some form of WOW or Care-Gram program (see Appendixes 9.9, 9.10 and 9.11). The point is simple: When you encourage employees to recognize each other for enhancing your patients' experience of care, they will respond by doing even better. Peer recognition increases staff's commitment to the job and to their patients. When peers recognize each other's commitment to patient satisfaction, the culture is reinforced. The result is more satisfied patients as well as employees.

Staff Are Regularly Evaluated for Their Patient Satisfaction Orientation

Staff are not only rewarded for success but are held accountable for decreases as well as increases in patient satisfaction scores. A portion of compensation may depend upon departmental or unit performance. Recognition that one's own performance can affect the compensation of one's peers is a powerful incentive. Part of job performance evaluations may include evaluations by staff in other departments or areas on the employee's ability to facilitate the tasks of others.

Staff Are Rewarded by Management for Their Commitment to Patient Satisfaction

Survey score increases are routinely praised and recognized. A minor budget item allows managers to distribute gift certificates (local fast-food restaurants will likely give you a bunch free) or other low-cost perks to their staff when scores go up. Returned surveys that praise specific staff members are posted publicly in that department. At JFK Medical Center in Edison, New Jersey, staff who receive five or more positive comments on patient satisfaction surveys during any data gathering period receive a "Superstar" pin from senior management. The pins are worn proudly.

Bonuses based on achieving specific patient satisfaction score goals may or may not be part of management strategy. It is not essential that you profit-share. Purely symbolic, nonmonetary rewards can be powerful incentives for maintaining the culture. At St. Luke's Episcopal Hospital in Houston, Texas, low ED satisfaction scores spurred a broadly supported QI effort. In the first quarter following project inception, the ED moved from the 5th to the 26th percentile among EDs in the Press Ganey national database. Even though this was still low-performing, St. Luke's president donned an apron and hosted an improvement-recognition party for ED staff. Within three quarters, St. Luke's ED had achieved 99th percentile status and were rewarded with a new stereo and automatic iced-tea maker for the staff lounge. These recognitions cost the hospital little but had significant effect on morale and commitment.

When Bristol Hospital in Bristol, Connecticut, hit the 95th percentile in the Press Ganey national patient satisfaction database, their CEO, Tom Kennedy, threw a lawn party and a cafeteria sundae celebration. Again, the cost is minimal but the impact great. The CEO's commitment is obvious.

CONCLUSIONS

All organizations have their special culture. Hospital cultures consist of all the roles, rules, behaviors, values, and opinions of staff and administration. Cultures are learned and transmitted via people observing and interacting with others, not through mission statements and edicts alone. The most effective patient satisfaction programs are institutionwide, reflecting commitment from the top to bottom. Otherwise, tension will be constant as committed elements run up against uncommitted departments or individuals who thwart the improvement processes. The goal is to make patient satisfaction such a part of the institutional culture that it is taken for granted. When formal programs are supplanted by everyday institutionwide behavioral demonstrations as the basic form of training, you have got your culture in place.

ACTION FOR SATISFACTION

1. Plan for an institutionwide, long-term program.
2. Make sure all staff play some role in improvement program planning and/or implementation.
3. Make patient satisfaction a mandatory meeting agenda item for all groups.
4. Emphasize patient satisfaction as a key criterion for employment, advancement, and reward. No staff group can be exempted.
5. Publicize patient satisfaction efforts and successes throughout the institution.
6. Develop general and specific scripting protocols.
7. Establish mechanisms for staff to reward each other for exemplary service.
8. Give regular, publicized rewards for exemplary or improved performance. Keep the fire burning.
9. Train and empower all staff to deal with service recovery.

REFERENCES

Cunningham, L., and M. P. Malone. 1999. "Newsletters Aren't Enough: Best Practices in Internal Communication Lead to Impressive Patient Satisfaction Scores." *Strategies for Healthcare Excellence* 12 (9): 1–7.

Eisenberg, B. 1997. "Customer Service in Healthcare: A New Era." *Hospital and Health Services Administration* 42 (1): 17–31.

Gutter, E., and M. Marinaro. 2002. "The Most Powerful Drug [Is Words]." *Satisfaction Monitor* (Jan/Feb): 1–3.

Mayer, T., and R. Cates. 2004. *Leadership for Great Customer Service: Satisfied Patients, Satisfied Employees.* Chicago: Health Administration Press.

Sherman, C. 1997. *Creating the New American Hospital.* San Francisco: Jossey-Bass.

Appendix 9.1. Covenant PRIDE Customer Satisfaction Welcome Letter

A message to the
PRIDE Customer Satisfaction
Team Members

We want to express our sincere appreciation and excitement for your participation in the Covenant PRIDE Customer Satisfaction program.

What you are about to read (and embark upon) was created by your peers – not executives sitting in an office far from the patient care front line. After talking with many of you, what we heard was that it was most important to you to be able to feel pride in the work you do because your work really matters to you.

The Covenant PRIDE program incorporates our Mission, Vision and Values into service standards, patient interaction guidelines and other elements of the PRIDE program that are outlined in this booklet. These are the "basics" for the strategy behind providing stellar care to our customers.

I strongly encourage you to have an open mind and give 100% as you embark on this program. We are indebted to you for helping us accomplish our goal of service excellence.

Chris Barnette
CHS Executive VP/Chief Operating Officer

CHS PRIDE Customer Satisfaction Vision Statement

We will be preferred and recognized for our values-based customer service by consistently achieving a patient satisfaction ranking in the top 10% of all hospitals our size.

Used with permission from Covenant Health System, Lubbock, Texas.

Appendix 9.2. Front Page of a Weekly Publication for the Employees of Bristol Hospital

Newsline

Volume XVII- No. 5 • **A Weekly Publication for the Employees of Bristol Hospital** *•*

From the President's Desk

Friday, our "Top 5% Patient Satisfaction Bonus Day," was a memorable day for me and I hope you share that feeling. I can report that 660 fellow employees came through the old ICU and received their cash bonus award. The other 245 bonus eligible employees will receive their compensation in the form of a check to be processed this week. Many of you took the time to thank me for what was happening on Friday. But the thanks really goes to you. Everyone who works here has contributed to our success under this program. If you want to thank someone, spread it around.

A number of employees asked me for more details about exactly what level of success we achieved. Over the course of the last nine months, we have been rated in the top 5%, which means we are better than 95 out of 100 hospitals in patient satisfaction. Given that within Press Ganey we compete against approximately 500 hospital who also are striving for excellence, this makes our achievement of top 5% very special. To put it simply, we are ranked as one of the top 20 hospitals in the Press Ganey universe.

We will be using every opportunity to boast about this significant achievement and all of your efforts in the newspaper and at the Home Show. The pride that I sense as I walk through the building is very real. I sense it not just among members of the work force, but also among our patients and their families. Our community is already responding with pride at our level of achievement.

On Friday we gave staff "Top 5%" blue ribbons to wear on their badge. These ribbons and window decals are for all employees. Stop by Public Relations on Level E if you do not yet have a ribbon or window decal. For at least the next month you may

proudly wear the ribbon in celebration of our accomplishment. I have every confidence that we can keep up this great work.

If your weekend allows, please come by the Bristol Hospital displays at the Chamber's Home Show. We would love to see you there.

- Tom Kennedy

Weekly Statistics (1/31/99 - 2/6/99)	
Admissions	
Budget:	135
Actual:	153
Last Year:	157
Patient Days	
Budget:	600
Actual:	574
Last Year:	725
Average Daily Census	
Budget:	86
Actual:	82
Last Year:	104
Outpatient Services (Reg.)	
Actual:	3630
Last Year:	3928

Congratulations to Both!

Many of you may have seen the article in *The Bristol Press* about EMT William Kenney. In addition to his duties here at Bristol Hospital, Bill is a 15 year veteran of the Bristol Police Department. He was recently chosen to be the 1999 Police Officer of the Year by the Exchange Club and will be honored at a dinner to be held at Nuchie's Restaurant on February 22. Joanne Kuntz, MD, will be the keynote speaker. One of his many accomplishments is being the motivating force in bringing automated defibrillators to the Bristol Police Department.

For those of you who wish to attend the dinner, tickets are available at the Bristol Police Department , Shannon's Jewelers and the Greater

Bristol Chamber of Commerce. Congratulations to Bill on this well-deserved honor.

Shirley Breuer, MA, PT, OCS, CSCS of Rehab Dynamics/ Newington was recently certified as a clinical specialist in orthopaedic physical therapy by the American Board of Physical Therapy Specialists. Shirley is one of 1245 physical therapists certified in the United States and one of 30 certified in the state of Connecticut. To receive board certification, candidates must successfully complete an extensive examination and demonstrate specialized knowledge and advanced clinical proficiency in a special area of physical therapy practice. Congratulations to Shirley on this most significant accomplishment.

Y2K - Squash the Bug
Personal Tips

The American Red Cross advises that you examine your smoke alarms now. If you have smoke alarms that are hardwired into your home's electrical system, check to see if they have battery back-ups. Every fall, replace all batteries in all smoke alarms.

Indemnity Dental Announcement

Effective February 1, 1999, a new company called The Phoenix will process your indemnity dental claims. **Your dental benefits have not changed**. Please use the forms being mailed to your home to submit claims incurred after 2-1-99 to The Phoenix. New dental ID cards will be issued by the end of February. Additional dental claim forms are available in the Human Resources Department.

(over)

Used with permission from Bristol Hospital, Bristol, Connecticut.

Appendix 9.3. Front Page of Columbus Regional Hospital's Newsletter, "In the Know"

In The Know at Columbus Regional Hospital

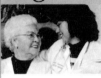

Know Your Customer...

Upcoming Activities

August 23 – 27 – Employee Photos Taken

August 25 – Satisfaction Fair

August 28 – Volunteer Day for Housing Partnerships

September 1 - Employee Update Session

September 4 - Hospice Concert

September 7 - Deadline to Register for Seven Habits

September 8 – Employee Picnic

COLUMBUS
REGIONAL
HOSPITAL

Satisfaction Fair
Visit the East Gallery on Wednesday, August 25th from 8 a.m. - 5:30 p.m. for the hospital's first-ever Satisfaction Fair. Over 30 booths will be set up for departments to share how they are working to improve customer satisfaction. Prizes will be awarded and special activities are planned. Come join the fun. Watch for next Wednesday's In The Know for a review of the event.

Extraordinary Story
The following is this month's Extraordinary Story which demonstrates hospital employees who are going the extra mile to deliver outstanding customer service for a fellow coworker...

When a sudden family crisis left Caroline McDaniel without childcare for her infant son, coworkers stepped in and volunteered to use their days off work to help out. "I was working nights and was not only struggling with child care during the night but also needed help during the day so I could rest. I could not have survived during this trying time without the help of my co-workers, and the support of my manager. I would like to recognize all 3 Tower employees for being patient with me during this difficult time. Special thanks to Brenda Murray, Anna Bunch, DeAnna Followell, Heather Welchel, Erica Jones, Beth Wright, Erin Haufe and Heather Haufe. Their commitment to me strengthened my commitment toward the hospital.

Weekly Satisfaction Score
The hospital's overall inpatient satisfaction score for the week of August 16th was a mean score of 82.8. The distribution of responses for the week was: Very Good 46%, Good 43%, Fair 10%, Poor 2%, Very Poor 0%. There has been a drop in Very Good responses down to Good, which has caused a decline in scores over the past few weeks. Continue to ask the question, "Is there anything else I can do for you?" as a way to help make a patient's experience very good.

Picnic Trivia
Q.   What movie was Walt Disney's first full-length animated film?

Read Friday's In The Know for the answer and a new movie trivia question to help prepare you for the movie-theme Employee Picnic on Wednesday, September 8th. The movie trivia question on Monday was, "Which movie was the top-grossing film at the box office last week?" Answer is "The Sixth Sense." Watch In The Know for more details about picnic activities.

Appendix 9.4. Pledge to Patient Satisfaction Required of All Bristol Hospital Staff

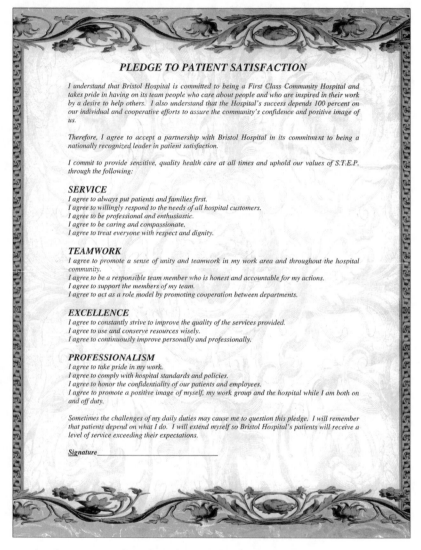

PLEDGE TO PATIENT SATISFACTION

I understand that Bristol Hospital is committed to being a First Class Community Hospital and takes pride in having on its team people who care about people and who are inspired in their work by a desire to help others. I also understand that the Hospital's success depends 100 percent on our individual and cooperative efforts to assure the community's confidence and positive image of us.

Therefore, I agree to accept a partnership with Bristol Hospital in its commitment to being a nationally recognized leader in patient satisfaction.

I commit to provide sensitive, quality health care at all times and uphold our values of S.T.E.P. through the following:

SERVICE
I agree to always put patients and families first.
I agree to willingly respond to the needs of all hospital customers.
I agree to be professional and enthusiastic.
I agree to be caring and compassionate.
I agree to treat everyone with respect and dignity.

TEAMWORK
I agree to promote a sense of unity and teamwork in my work area and throughout the hospital community.
I agree to be a responsible team member who is honest and accountable for my actions.
I agree to support the members of my team.
I agree to act as a role model by promoting cooperation between departments.

EXCELLENCE
I agree to constantly strive to improve the quality of the services provided.
I agree to use and conserve resources wisely.
I agree to continuously improve personally and professionally.

PROFESSIONALISM
I agree to take pride in my work.
I agree to comply with hospital standards and policies.
I agree to honor the confidentiality of our patients and employees.
I agree to promote a positive image of myself, my work group and the hospital while I am both on and off duty.

Sometimes the challenges of my daily duties may cause me to question this pledge. I will remember that patients depend on what I do. I will extend myself so Bristol Hospital's patients will receive a level of service exceeding their expectations.

<u>Signature</u>_____

Used with permission from Bristol Hospital, Bristol, Connecticut.

Appendix 9.5. Expectations of Baptist Health System Staff

BAPTIST EXPECTATIONS

Baptist Health Systems is an organization that is committed to our heritage, superior customer service and dedication to the Christian healing ministry. This is reflected in all contacts with our patients, visitors, physicians and fellow team members. Our commitment is to provide First Class customer service and we will accept nothing less. To that end, our employees are dedicated to the following expectations:

- Every individual is uniquely created and deserves special attention and recognition.

- Every employee is totally committed to being a valued team player.

- Every employee is expected to be a First Class ambassador for Baptist Health Systems.

- Every employee is empowered and has resources to satisfy and impress our customers.

- Every employee is expected to respond promptly to opportunities which will meet the needs of our customers.

- Every employee is expected to be at work when scheduled and on time.

- Every employee is expected to follow the personal appearance guidelines and present themselves in a professional manner at all times.

- Every employee takes pride in excellence, looks for opportunities for improvement and views problems as opportunities.

- Every employee is expected to perform their job to the best of their abilities.

As a future employee of Baptist Health Systems, I understand and am willing to commit to these stated expectations.

Name: _____   Date: _____

HR-067
(11-10-99)

Used with permission from Baptist Health Systems, Jackson, Mississippi.

Appendix 9.6. Covenant Health System's PRIDE Customer Service Standards

IV. PRIDE Customer Service Standards

Covenant
Health System

Service

We bring together people who recognize that every interaction is a unique opportunity to serve one another, the community, and society.

CUSTOMER/PATIENT FOCUS (Values-Based Competency)
- Anticipate and strive to understand the unique needs of those serving as well as those served.
- Respond to the needs of those served and demonstrate concern for meeting those needs.
- Tailor each interaction to the specific needs of the person and/or situation.

★ ★ ★ ★ ★ ★ ★ ★
SERVICE STANDARD 9

Anticipate the wants and needs of those served.

- Be aware of and sensitive to the different cultures and religious beliefs of others.
- If delays are anticipated, communicate it to the patient. If there are delays do not place blame – NEVER SAY *"We are short-staffed."*
- Be sensitive to patient needs such as hearing impairments, language barriers and disabilities.
- Focus on the education, comfort and privacy needs of patients before, during and after treatments and procedures.
- Always provide patients with blankets during transports to ensure warmth and dignity.
- Survey the patient environment and be sure to ask if there is anything you can provide to make them more comfortable.
- Listen. When people complain, don't be defensive. Hear them out and show understanding. Do all you can to make things right.
- Put the patient and family at ease. Reach out with friendly words and gestures.
- Show concern for the well being of others.

★ ★ ★ ★ ★ ★ ★ ★

CHS PRIDE Customer Satisfaction Vision Statement

We will be preferred and recognized for our values-based customer service by consistently achieving a patient satisfaction ranking in the top 10% of all hospitals our size.

Used with permission from Covenant Health System, Lubbock, Texas.

Appendix 9.7. The Beaumont Standards

The Beaumont Standards

The Beaumont Standards will be known, owned and energized by all Beaumont employees.

Service

Wait times – Make every effort to provide prompt service.
- Apologize for any delay in service.
- When a delay occurs, update patients regarding their status at least every 20 minutes.
- Once service is rendered, thank patients for waiting.
- Update family members at least hourly when patients undergo a procedure.
- When interruptions occur while providing service to patients, complete their service first before moving on.
- Ask permission before placing telephone callers on hold; thank them for their patience when you return to the telephone.

Information - Provide clear explanations and accurate information.
- Explain what service you will be providing and what to expect next.

Response - Respond promptly to those requesting service.
- If you cannot perform the requested service immediately, provide a time frame for completion.
- If a request for service cannot be completed by you, refer it to the person who can.
- Answer telephone calls within three rings.
- When answering the telephone, identify your department, yourself and ask, "How may I help you?"
- If a patient's call light goes on, anyone is responsible to respond regardless of job classification.
- Respond to call lights with, "How may I help you?"
- Inform your patients when you will be away for a break or meal and when you expect to return.

Ownership

Directions – Offer to escort others who appear lost and need assistance.
- Personally escort lost people to their destination or find someone who can.
- When giving directions with hand gestures, use two-finger or full-hand gestures.

Teamwork – Show your pride in being part of the Beaumont team.
- Be a positive ambassador of the hospital in what you say and do.
- Pick up litter and report spills.
- Return all items or equipment to their proper place.

Attitude

Image – Observe the highest standards of grooming; dress professionally as appropriate to your discipline.
- Wear your Beaumont ID badge exposed at all times, either in the breast pocket area or on a provided ID badge necklace.
- Dress according to dress code.

Courtesy – Project the image that you are eager to help and that serving others is never an interruption.
- Respond with expressions such as "certainly," "I'd be happy to" or "my pleasure."
- When transporting patients in wheelchairs, face them toward the elevator door.
- Offer to exit an elevator or wait for another elevator so patients on stretchers may be transported first.
- End service interactions with, "Is there anything else I can do for you? I have time."

Respect

Introduction - Introduce yourself by name and function.
- Acknowledge others with a verbal greeting, eye contact and appropriate gestures.
- Smile and introduce yourself by your name and function.
- Address patients and families by their name and appropriate title (e.g. Mr., Mrs.) unless invited to use a more familiar name.

Confidentiality – Hold all patient and employee information in the highest confidence.
- Access only information that is essential to your job.
- When discussing sensitive matters, seek a private location.

Dignity – Provide privacy, respect cultural and spiritual values.
- Knock or ask permission before entering.
- Close doors and curtains during examinations, procedures and interviews.
- Provide a robe or second gown to ambulating patients and cover patients being transported.
- Make sure gowns are the right size for patients.
- Affirm patients' rights to make choices regarding their care.

Beaumont®
William Beaumont Hospital

Used with permission from William Beaumont Hospital, Troy, Michigan.

Appendix 9.8. William Beaumont Hospital's Performance Standards Commitment

William Beaumont Hospital
Troy

Performance Standards Commitment
William Beaumont Hospital, Troy

I have read and understand the Performance Standards that were developed by William Beaumont Hospital, Troy employees, and understand they are a measure of work performance. They are printed on cards to be attached to my identification badge and were attached to this document.

I understand by incorporating these standards as a measure of work performance, William Beaumont Hospital leadership makes it clear that we are all accountable for adhering to and practicing these standards.

I further understand that these standards apply equally to the interactions between all customer groups – patients, families, physicians and each other.

As a member of the William Beaumont Hospital, Troy Team, I am committed to the Standards and agree to not only hold myself accountable for doing so, but also to expect the same from all other Beaumont staff.

_____
Employee Signature

_____
Employee Name *(Please print)*   **ID #**

_____
Department

_____
Date

Used with permission from William Beaumont Hospital, Troy, Michigan.

Appendix 9.9. Baptist Health Care's WOW Card

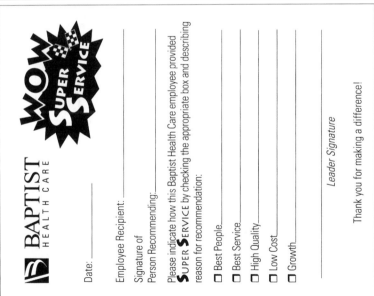

The mission of Baptist Health Care is to provide superior service based on Christian values to improve the quality of life for people and communities served.

Living the values and **Exceeding** the Standards to **Achieve** our vision of making Baptist Health Care the **Best** health system in America.

BAPTIST HEALTH CARE

Attitude
Appearance
Communication
Call Lights
Commitment to Co-Workers
Customer Waiting
Elevator Etiquette
Privacy
Safety Awareness
Sense of Ownership

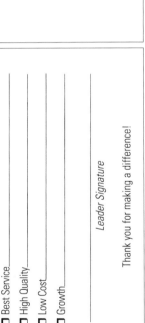

BAPTIST HEALTH CARE

WOW SUPER SERVICE

Date: _____

Employee Recipient: _____

Signature of
Person Recommending: _____

Please indicate how this Baptist Health Care employee provided
SUPER **S**ERVICE by checking the appropriate box and describing
reason for recommendation:

☐ Best People _____
☐ Best Service _____
☐ High Quality _____
☐ Low Cost _____
☐ Growth _____

_____
Leader Signature

Thank you for making a difference!

Used with permission from Baptist Health Care Corporation, Pensacola, Florida.

Appendix 9.10. Bristol Hospital's WOW Certificate

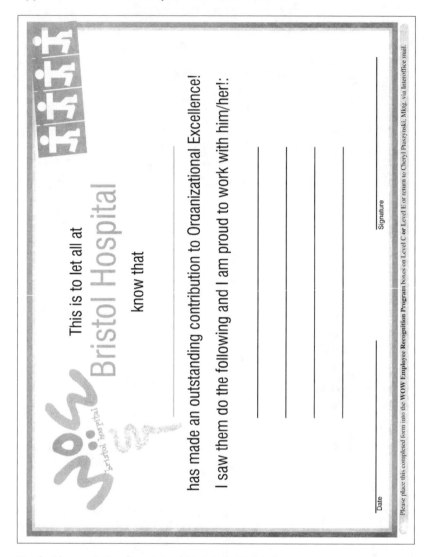

Used with permission from Bristol Hospital, Bristol, Connecticut.

Appendix 9.11. Kern Medical Center's Tell-A-Gram

Tell-A-Gram

The Tell-A-Gram acknowledges a special act of customer service. It is an expression of "going the extra mile".

Have you seen an employee(s) or department demonstrate a special act of service toward a customer or co-worker? Has someone done something to make your time pleasant or comfortable? Has a co-worker helped to make your job a little bit easier?

If the answer is yes, please acknowledge this example of commitment to outstanding customer service by giving that person (or department) a Tell-A-Gram.

Anyone may give a Tell-A-Gram - patient, customer, volunteer, employee, vendor, visitor, or guest.

Simply fill out the reverse side of this card and briefly describe the special act which deserves recognition. Then, place the card in the specially designated Tell-A-Gram boxes or mail to:

KMC Human Resources
1830 Flower Street
Bakersfield, CA 93305

We will make sure the Tell-A-Gram is delivered to the person, their supervisor and the Customer Service Task Force.

Thank you for your participation!

KERN MEDICAL CENTER

Tell-A-Gram
a great way to say thank you

5917-3075 (4/98)

Recipient: _____
First and Last Name (One card per person or department)

Name of Department: _____

Date Service Performed: _____

Time Observed: _____

This person has provided outstanding customer service in the following way:

_____
_____
_____
_____
_____
_____
_____
_____

Please print your name and telephone number (required).

Name _____ Phone _____

Used with permission from Kern Medical Center, Bakersfield, California.

From Action to Satisfaction—Creating a Culture, Not Just a Program   199

CHAPTER 10

Fifty Nifty Ideas for Improving Patient Satisfaction

*Mary Malone**

YOU DO NOT have to spend big bucks or big time to improve your patients' experience. It does not require a grand event or program to wow them. Gentle, symbolic gestures can create very positive patient perceptions of the staff and hospital as friendly, caring, empathetic, and competent. This is not trivial. Anything that allays the patient's anxiety and contributes to trust also contributes to the effectiveness and evaluation of care. When a nurse slips an empty Starbuck's coffee sack over the IV bag of a patient who is not yet allowed anything by mouth, it reflects a wry empathy that says, "I know how you must feel. I know you want your coffee. I know you want normalcy." Here, a simple gesture links patient and nurse as collaborators in understanding the personal impact of the medical problem and its treatment.

Here are a bunch of ideas—most of them easy and inexpensive —that can make a difference to patients.

---

* Mary Malone, M.S., J.D., is president of Malone Advisory Services. She previously spent nearly 15 years at Press Ganey Associates, where she served as executive director of consulting services. Mary consults widely for hospitals across the country, focusing on patient satisfaction and process improvement.

FIRST IMPRESSIONS AND WELCOMING EXPERIENCES

Every healthcare encounter has a beginning, middle, and end. First impressions are important for setting the tone for the organization and for the individual employee who is delivering care.

1. While going through an automated telephone tree to get to the right extension seems commonplace, at Wright Patterson Air Force Base Medical Center (74th Medical Group) in Dayton, Ohio, none other than the Commander (CEO) gives the welcome and introduces the phone menu.

2. Adapting a concept first used at Wal-Mart, many hospitals have added greeters at the front door to provide general informational and other types of assistance. At Vanderbilt University Medical Center in Nashville, Tennessee, greeters are armed with PDAs, and they check in ambulatory surgery patients so that when the patients arrive in the ambulatory surgery area, the staff has already been informed that they are there. This is not registration; it is merely a check-in that notifies the staff that the patient has arrived.

3. While implementing a "key words at key times" scripting strategy, many organizations have focused on the first impressions created at the change of shift and have implemented specific greetings for caregivers to give to patients and families at the beginning of their shift. This is also a continuity of care issue.

4. Among many successful strategies to welcome patients, Baptist Health Care in Pensacola, Florida, includes the CEOs home telephone number in patients' welcome packets, sending a powerful message of both his confidence in the hospital staff and willingness to be accessible to patients and families.

5. Northwestern Memorial Hospital in Chicago, Illinois, and the University of Chicago Hospitals provide "baseball cards" to patients and families, showing the names and pictures of the

physicians (usually the hospitalists) who are responsible for the patients' care. Other organizations, including the Mayo Clinic, place large photos of the attending physicians and residents who are working on the unit in a centralized area accessible to staff and patients alike.

6. At CentraState Medical Center in Freehold, New Jersey, one ED physician became known as the "pillow doc" because he always brought a pillow with him, saying "I thought this might make you feel more comfortable" whenever he met a new a patient. Patients consistently report being delighted by the extra attention to their physical needs.

7. If you happen to be walking by Sharp Coronado Hospital in Coronado, California, as many community members do each day, then stop in the lobby and grab a homemade chocolate chip cookie. Employees volunteer to make them to keep the lobby stocked and to encourage people to drop by the hospital, even when they are not sick.

8. Nurses at St. Joseph Medical Center in Kansas City, Missouri (part of Carondelet Health System), implemented a program called First Touch(TM) in their cardiac step-down unit. One of the objectives of the program is to initiate a conversation with the patient about the patient before touching or doing anything clinical—to have the first touch be one of person-to-person contact. This has extended into hellos and goodbyes, as well as improving transitions and handoffs between staff members, especially at shift change.

9. Many organizations, among them Westchester Medical Group in White Plains, New York, and the Mayo Clinic in Rochester, Minnesota, are experimenting with using kiosks to check in patients and complete the registration process. Like the greeters mentioned previously, the purpose is to notify staff of the patient's arrival. In this case, it is an automated setup. Patients can insert a credit card or other scanable ID. It is quick and efficient. With special software, functions can include the ability to have patients complete consent forms, acknowledge

receipt of HIPAA privacy guidelines, and pay for co-pays and outstanding balances.

10. The Diagnostic Center at the University of Texas M. D. Anderson Cancer Center in Houston, Texas, wanted to put a positive spin on their patient's days, even though the day sometimes starts with an uncomfortable blood draw. To take their minds off the procedure, the staff created Inspiration Alley—hanging inspirational poems and reflections within the line of sight of patients in the blood drawing area. The pieces are so popular with patients that staff soon hung baskets with copies of the sayings underneath the frames, and patients are encouraged to take copies home with them.

LASTING IMPRESSIONS AND POWERFUL GOODBYES

Every patient encounter has an ending, which provides a final opportunity to create a memorable experience for patients and to resolve any outstanding service issues.

11. In addition to post-discharge phone calls made to patients' homes, some ambulatory surgery centers and surgical nursing units mail thinking-of-you cards signed by all members of the caregiving (clinicians and non-clinicians) team to patients' homes upon their discharge. This is a great idea because it jogs patients' memories about their care and who attended them. This makes it more likely that patients will mention specific staff when filling out their satisfaction surveys. It provides more opportunity for staff to feel recognized and appreciated.

12. A number of oncology departments, including Thibodoux Regional Medical Center in Thibodoux, Louisiana, have developed meaningful ceremonies for patients completing rounds of chemotherapy or radiation treatments. Cardiac rehab programs have graduation ceremonies—complete with

caps and gowns—for patients who have completed their programs.

13. Spartanburg Hospital for Restorative Care in Spartanburg, South Carolina, plans elaborate celebrations for its patients who are being discharged, often after very lengthy stays in the rehab facility. For many patients with devastating injuries, returning home may once have seemed out of the question. Themed parties are planned, with appropriate musical accompaniment such as Roy Roger's *Happy Trails* and Willie Nelson's *On the Road Again*, and the patient's healing and rehabilitative and life accomplishments are celebrated.

14. Occasionally, patients at a number of hospitals will have the unique experience of being escorted from the lobby to their cars by the hospital CEO and other senior executives who are "rounding on patients" in public areas of their facilities.

15. More than 200 volunteers, including many from the hospital staff at Sacred Heart Medical Center in Eugene, Oregon, participate in the No One Dies Alone program. These employees—from all departments of the organization—are on-call to volunteer (day or night) to come and sit with a dying patient who has no one else to be there.

THE DISCHARGE PROCESS AS A LAST IMPRESSION

Getting home from the hospital, even after the patient has been told to expect to go home, can be a frustrating experience. Problems related to the discharge process can also have negative ramifications for the flow of patients and capacity issues throughout the entire organization.

16. Baptist Memorial Hospital in Memphis, Tennessee, does not simply schedule discharges by the day, morning, or evening. It schedules discharges by the quarter-hour (e.g., 9 a.m., 9:15

a.m.). They also use discharge checklists to help make sure the patient is ready at the specified time. This improves room availability and, more importantly, gives patients a greater feeling of control.

17. Getting all of the necessary educational information, discharge instructions, discharge orders, prescriptions, and supplies together for a patient's discharge is often time-consuming and disorganized. Patients are bombarded with information, and the process can seem disorienting and disjointed for patients, families, physicians, and nurses. One physician at South Bend Orthopedic Associates in South Bend, Indiana, has created an innovative and time-saving process for his patients. At their final office visit *prior* to elective surgery, patients are given discharge instructions, prescriptions for pain medicine, and a list of supplies for caring for their incisions. Following their surgery, the actual discharge process takes less than five minutes, during which staff check to make sure the patient has what he or she needs.

AMENITIES AND SPECIAL SERVICES

Little extras that make patients feel better or provide an unexpected pleasant surprise are growing in popularity. Many of them are low-cost or no-cost ideas. For those that have small associated costs, hospital auxiliaries have often stepped in to make donations to cover the expense.

18. A church group in Hollywood, Florida, crochets lap covers, blankets, and shawls for patients hospitalized at Memorial Regional Hospital. Patients are encouraged to take these special items home with them.

19. At the Hospital for Special Surgery in New York, New York, amenity packets for patients who may wait in the

post-anesthesia care unit (PACU) for an available inpatient bed include the standard toiletries and a tiny transistor radio and earphone.

20. New moms at a number of hospitals in the Midwest, including North Kansas City Hospital in North Kansas City, Missouri, receive library cards for their baby upon discharge. This is a neat image-enhancing act.

21. At Great River Medical Center in West Burlington, Iowa, volunteer storywriters capture and create a living history for long-term patients and those with chronic diseases requiring multiple hospitalizations. All caregivers (clinical and non-clinical) read about the patients' life stories, not only their medical histories, to learn about who the patients are and not only what diseases they have.

22. Waterbury Hospital in Waterbury, Conneticut, is among several providers that have worked as sponsors with their local newspapers and businesses to provide free newspapers for delivery to patient rooms, visitor lounges, and waiting areas.

23. To address patients' spiritual needs, a phone line can be set aside for a daily devotion, meditation, or prayer. At some organizations, these phone lines are also equipped to take incoming messages, such as requests for a visit from the hospital chaplain.

24. Sometimes, it is the small things that help patients prepare for surgery. The surgical prep team at Sharp Mary Birch Hospital for Women in San Diego, California, serves the iced, preoperative antacid in a shot glass, with a little mermaid and plastic umbrella hanging off the side. Other organizations serve post-procedure beverages in a fancy martini glass on a silver tray.

25. The surgical prep team in the ambulatory area at St. Joseph's Hospital in Chewaleh, Washington, understands that patients may arrive NPO (i.e., "nothing by mouth") and missing their morning coffee. To help lighten the moment, the staff will use an empty, one-pound coffee sack and place it over the

IV bag, giving the impression that the patient is getting their morning coffee in an unusual way. In a lighthearted way, this also expresses empathy with the patient's discomfort.

FOOD AND NUTRITION SERVICES

There are many ways in which food services can create positive impressions for the patient and their families. Room service and individualized menus are already found in a number of hospitals. Here are some other ideas.

26. Highland Park Hospital in Highland Park, Illinois, and Edward Hospital in Naperville, Illinois, in conjunction with their food service contract management company, have developed a program of utilizing local chefs and restaurateurs to cook meals for patients once a month. Meals are prepared for a wide range of diet types, giving most patients a chance to enjoy the special event.

27. Local chefs are also being used in growing numbers to teach heart-healthy eating and to demonstrate recipes in diabetes and cardiac education programs for patients and in community education programs and classes. Favorite local recipes are also prepared for patients, and the recipe cards are delivered on patient trays with their meals.

28. Kaiser Permanente medical centers in California, Colorado, and Utah encourage healthy eating among patients and employees by regularly hosting a farmer's market filled with local produce. The market is located in their parking lot. It is a great image enhancer for the hospital and a convenience for staff.

29. A combination of restaurant-style menus, room service (including meals for visitors), and/or enhanced retail services (e.g., cafeterias, cafés, coffee shops, nationally branded kiosks) have become commonplace in most organizations. Some food service departments use mobile carts to bring refreshments

to patient/family waiting areas, lobbies, and EDs. Typically, beverages may be gratis, with nominal charges for food. The mobile carts also make the rounds of nursing units, where busy nurses and caregivers (who may be unable to leave the unit for a trip to the cafeteria) can purchase a sandwich, soup, snacks, or a beverage.

IMPROVING COMMUNICATION AND INVOLVING FAMILY MEMBERS

One part of the patient's hospital experience that is easily overlooked is the family. Spouses, children, and parents are often more aware and critical of what is happening than their loved ones. Family members' interpretations of events and comments to the patient have an impact on the patient's perception and evaluation of care—both during and after the hospitalization. When families are integrated into the care through adequate communication, both the patient and hospital have an important ally. Later, when the satisfaction survey arrives at the house, few patients complete them in isolation from the family's input.

30. Patients, their family members and friends, as well as intensive care nurses and physicians have reaped benefits from eliminating traditional visiting hours from ICUs. Geisinger Medical Center in Danville, Pennsylvania, has been among the leaders in the open–visiting hours movement.
31. Interdisciplinary rounds among hospital staff have been met with widespread approval from clinicians and have resulted in significant improvements in quality. A new twist on interdisciplinary rounds is to include the patient and family as active participants in the team, discussing the care plan and short-term and long-term clinical goals. While this is a relatively new practice, it represents a significant departure from traditional rounding practice, where the patient and family are largely peripheral.

32. A number of hospitals encourage patients and their families to ask questions by including a pad and paper—often with the prompter, "What questions do you have for us?" as a heading—as part of the welcome packet that patients receive upon admission.

33. Thunderbird Samaritan Medical Center in Glendale, Arizona, has developed an extensive Partners in Caring program. Patients designate a "care partner," who is invited to be an important part of the care team. The partner receives a special name badge and a welcome packet with ideas for helping the patient and for personal stress reduction, and is encouraged to be involved in and assist with the patient's care and recovery.

34. At Centra Health in Lynchburg, Virginia, nurses leave voicemail messages with patient updates on the hospital's phone system twice a day. Family members, including those that live far away, can call into the voicemail box and receive an update about a loved one's condition. The hospital avoids HIPAA privacy concerns by furnishing an access code to the patient's designated care partner, who is then responsible for its dissemination.

35. A number of hospitals have service standards for ICU staff that include visits to patients within 24 hours of their being transferred to other units. The idea is to "see how they are doing" and to generally make another connection with them. At Baptist Memorial Hospital in Memphis, Tennessee, these transition visits have a clinical function as well; the ICU float charge nurse will assess the patient and intervene as necessary.

WAITING TIMES AND CALL-BUTTON RESPONSE

Considered by many patients to be the bane of their healthcare experiences, the nature of the business may mean that some waits are inevitable. However, much is being done to reduce waits and the stress and anxiety that are associated with them.

36. Significant reductions in patient waits are being accomplished using process improvement techniques (e.g., Six Sigma, Lean Engineering) that focus workflow processes. In many departments, quality improvement activities that dramatically increase the number of appointments, procedures, and surgeries that start on time also prevent waiting time buildup during the day. Improvements in scheduling processes use historical data to determine likely numbers of emergencies and to schedule an estimated number of emergency slots throughout the day, thus preventing patient backlogs. When waiting times occasionally occur, more advanced strategies range from giving patients restaurant-style beepers if waits are going to be excessive to having a physicians' office with schedules that only offer same-day appointments. The beeper system typically allows patients and family to roam rather than be forced to sit in a waiting room.

37. A bold statement about eliminating waits was made during the design process for the new ED at Ball Memorial Hospital in Muncie, Indiana (part of Cardinal Health). It was designed and constructed without a waiting room. Space that would have been used for the waiting room was utilized instead for additional treatment rooms that are large enough to include family members or friends who accompanied the patient to the ED.

38. Perception matters in small ways as well. A waiting room is for waiting. Creative organizations are renaming waiting areas with different functions in mind: hospitality area, resource center, family center, or reception area. This not only changes patient expectations about the space but also changes how the organization approaches the ways in which patients and others will use their time in the space.

39. Rather than provide old magazines, some organizations, including the Mayo Clinic in Rochester, Minnesota, place

jigsaw puzzles on tables for patients and visitors to complete. Some medical practices have a cookbook collection, such as low-fat cooking at a cardiology practice, with index cards and pens nearby. The recipes make interesting reading (and perhaps writing) and never go out of date.

40. Other techniques used in physician waiting rooms and other hospitality areas to create positive distractions for patients during waits include collage pictures of the physicians and office staff in seasonal garb, guess-whose-baby-picture contests, rotating wall art with other physician offices or public library collections, aquariums, and terrariums. In larger lobbies, waiting patients, family members, and staff often enjoy piano music— sometimes scheduled concerts, sometimes impromptu playing by a willing volunteer.

41. Waiting for a call-button response is a particularly frustrating experience for patients. But the available research shows that most call-button needs are relatively predictable—pain, potty, and position. A group of 22 hospitals participating in the Alliance for Health Care Research has been working to significantly reduce the number of times patients need to use call buttons. Many strategies were employed. Regular, hourly anticipatory rounds as well as standard assessments of room setups and environmental assessments by *all* staff entering or leaving the patient's room were among the most successful.

SERVICE GUARANTEES

Perhaps the ultimate expression of a commitment to service excellence, service guarantees are not yet widely employed in the healthcare setting. But they make an impressive statement to customers, employees, and the community alike.

42. CHRISTUS Health (an integrated delivery system headquartered in Irving, Texas) advertises a service guarantee

at all its facilities throughout Texas, Louisiana, and nearby states. The guarantee focuses on prompt attention, honest communication, and attention to special needs. These are not difficult to provide, and the guarantee makes a very positive impression on patients and their families.

43. Hospitals throughout New Jersey, including those affiliated with the Robert Wood Johnson Health System and Network, have service guarantees for their EDs. Patients will see a nurse within 15 minutes and a physician within 30 minutes of their arrival, or the hospital will not bill for the visit.

EMPLOYEES AND PHYSICIANS

Successful service organizations recognize that positive employee and physician experiences are essential to delivering their service promises. Innovative ideas to engage and satisfy these constituencies are becoming more popular among leading organizations.

44. A week or two before beginning employment at Centegra Health System in Woodstock, Illinois, new employees should not be surprised if they receive a phone call from the hospital's president and CEO to welcome them to his team.

45. As a unique twist on the celebration and recognition evening for long-tenured employees (i.e., 25 years or more), the human resources department at Ingalls Memorial Hospital in Harvey, Illinois, shares a copy of the employee's original job application and some thought-provoking questions as conversation starters (e.g., Where were you living at the time? What type of car were you driving? What music were you listening to?).

46. Froedtert Hospital in Milwaukee, Wisconsin, has an unusual and highly successful strategy for nurse staffing. In general, nurses at the hospital are scheduled for one of two schedules: A or B. The A nurses work one week, Monday–Sunday, for ten hours every day and then have the next seven days off.

The B team nurses have the first week off and then work the second Monday–Sunday schedule. (Froedtert also uses an overlap system that concentrates nurses on the unit from noon until late afternoon.) The A and B weeks are known years in advance, and staff can easily plan time-off and vacations. The unusual schedule is popular and a factor in the organization's very low turnover and vacancy rates compared to national and state averages.

47. Achieving higher volumes—whether inpatient census, ED visits, or procedure-counts—play an important role in healthcare strategic plans. But from a staff perspective, increased volume can seem like just more work. A number of hospitals have taken to providing simple rewards, such as a cafeteria visit for all employees, on days when the census exceeds targeted levels.

48. Employees at some hospitals benefit from the concierge services provided by their organizations. This is growing in popularity as a recruiting and retention strategy. Among the services that are offered are dry cleaning service drop-off and pick-up; car services such as oil changes or car washes; and an expanded gift shop that is also a convenience store, with items such as milk, bread, and kid's school project supplies. Late-shifters find this especially helpful, as do patients and families.

49. Spartanburg Regional Healthcare System in Spartanburg, South Carolina, took nurse scheduling to new levels when they pioneered an online auction for working shifts. An employee can submit a bid to work a shift at $45 per hour and another employee can submit a lower bid, such as $43 per hour; the process continues until the auction closes. Employees have greater access to picking up a shift within their own institution, and the organization wins with better-qualified staff and costs that are less than using an agency or contract nurses. Increasingly, hospitals are taking advantage of information technology to improve and streamline scheduling systems and permit more units to use self-scheduling to cover shifts.

50. A Doctor's Week celebrations at one hospital included a hallway filled with survey quotes from patients and families recognizing the physicians on cutout stars. At the conclusion of the week, the stars were gathered up and sent to the physicians' homes so their family members could join in the celebration as well.

CONCLUSIONS

These are not earth-shattering ideas. They demonstrate the possibilities of imagination and, in many instances, zero-based budgeting, where concepts such as "this is the way it's always been done" are tossed out the window. Serving meds in a shot glass with an umbrella is admittedly hokey, but it is effective because it expresses a connection with the patient's discomfort. Small, isolated, unexpected but positive experiences can have a powerful impact on patients' perceptions of care. Patient satisfaction derives from the collective impact of largely symbolic experiences, not expensive new wings or EDs.

CHAPTER 11

The Emergency Department:
A Special Case

PATIENT SATISFACTION IN the ED offers special challenges. The emergency encounter is brief, relatively speaking, and usually stressful. Establishing rapport is difficult. For many patients, the ED visit is their first experience with the hospital or medical center and its related services. This means that patients' ED experiences have major marketing implications. You may not be making a buck on the ED, but if patients decide they do not like your emergency facilities, then you will soon find your more profitable service revenues falling. Finally, patient and staff ideas of "emergency" may differ significantly. The nature of the emergency patient constituency is changing, and staff are frequently unprepared to face this new healthcare customer.

ARE THEY PATIENTS OR CUSTOMERS?

Caring, dedicated staff often have difficulty viewing patients as customers, yet the shifting nature of hospital care demands precisely such a perspective. As hospitals expand the range of services they offer to attract managed care contracts as well as patients in general, branding becomes important. Each year, about 20,000 to 70,000 patients pass through EDs. If patients are turned off by the experience, then they may opt not to use the hospital's operating room or physician practice (or birthing center or cardiac center or home health agency) later on. The opposite is true, too. If patients are highly satisfied with emergency care, then positive marketing has occurred. They will be more likely to select the hospital or its affiliated services for future care needs. Moreover, up to half of all inpatients are admitted through the ED. If patients are satisfied with the emergency experience, then they enter the hospital more positively predisposed toward inpatient care. This positive predisposition translates into greater collaboration and less likelihood of claims.

Do patients view themselves as customers?

We were surprised, as were Press Ganey's emergency survey clients, to discover that one of the items most highly correlated with the likelihood of patients recommending the ED to others is not a technical quality issue. Rather, it is the issue of value. Of all items on the emergency survey, one of those most highly related to satisfaction was whether the emergency care was worth the money charged.

Patients increasingly recognize that they are customers. Through insurance premiums, salary reductions, or co-pays, the majority are paying for emergency care one way or another—and they know it. They pay for everything else in their lives and have come to expect and demand both service and value.

Thom Mayer, president and CEO of Best Practices, Inc., says that they are both patients and customers (Mayer and Cates 2004). Some are almost all patient and more "horizontal" (i.e., very sick and very out of it). Some are mostly customer and conceptually more "vertical" (i.e., minimally sick, ambulatory, maximally aware of what is going on). Every patient is to some extent a customer.

One afternoon, I observed the following (from field notes):

A young mother (with insurance) brings her baby into the ED, stating that she accidentally spilled hot tea on her child's arm. Seeing only a slight bit of redness, the triage nurse makes the woman wait. Finally seen by a doctor, she is told that "there's nothing there" and that she "can put some salve on the baby's arm when you get home."

"What salve?" she asks.

"Any one you have at home," answers the doctor curtly.

The mother leaves, very upset. She angrily says, "My baby's arm is burned. After all this time waiting I'm only told to go home and put some salve on it? Any old salve? Maybe I have some salve at home, and maybe I don't! What kind of treatment is this?" Here, she feels that her baby has received insufficient and rather cavalier care. She is unaware, of course, that it takes just as much medical expertise to judge that nothing is wrong as to diagnose a real problem. She leaves feeling she has not gotten value for her money. She wants medical care. But she is clearly very much a customer for this care.

Mothers who bring their children into the ED are always 100 percent customer and 0 percent patient. Here is a positive example of a patient getting her money's worth (from field notes):

A 30-something woman presents with a complaint of having "burned my mouth while eating ice cream. I took a big bite and a huge glob of it stuck to the roof of my mouth." She feels somewhat embarrassed by the incident. The physician examines her and tells her that she must gargle with salt water every two hours for the remainder of the day. "Don't miss a single time," he admonishes. She leaves very satisfied. The doctor has taken her seriously and made her feel that her decision to come to this ED was proper.

Both of these women were a small percent patient and a large percent customer.

In Chapter 2, I mentioned a company that switched insurance plans because of some employees' dissatisfaction with their in-network hospital; it was largely ED experiences that triggered the defection. Now the company's growing staff use the ED, outpatient clinics, physician practices, and inpatient facilities of a competing hospital. Did the first hospital lose patients or customers?

WHO IS AN EMERGENCY PATIENT?

Many patients should not be in the ED—just ask your staff! Staff have yet to come to grips with the fact that perhaps half the patients are using the ED for primary care rather than strict emergencies. The U.S. government estimates that close to 55 percent of ED patients are nonurgent (McCaig 1994). A typical ED staff estimate this at closer to 75 percent.

The problem with categorizing patients as primary care versus real emergency lies with the definition and—more precisely—whose perspective is driving the definition. A new mother presents with her baby at 2:00 p.m., stating that her baby "didn't eat lunch." Staff eyes roll, and they think, "Another crock is here wasting our time." It is a good bet that she will be punished for presenting inappropriately by being made to wait. If a researcher subsequently were to use the medical records to do a study of ED use by emergent versus primary care patients, then the young mother would surely be defined as a primary care case. To her, however, the problem is an emergency, and staff do not seem to be taking her very seriously. She is still insecure with the responsibilities of motherhood and is frightened by the change in her new infant's eating pattern. To her, it is an emergency.

This can lead highly trained emergency professionals to feel abused by patients, especially during busy shifts. How easy is it to satisfy customers you feel are abusing you?

WHAT IS AN EMERGENCY?

In Chapter 3, we discussed patients and staff as representing two different cultures. This is certainly the case in the ED.

Differences in values and expectations begin with the very definition of emergency and the proper function of the ED. To staff, the ED's function is essentially to stabilize patients. To patients, the function is to heal, not merely to stabilize. Thus, the emergency encounter often begins with significant misunderstanding of its very purpose. What constitutes an emergency in the first place? Patients define a medical problem as an emergency when one or more of three thresholds are crossed:

1. *Threshold of discomfort*: The pain or discomfort is at an unbearable level.
2. *Threshold of anxiety*: The condition causes such anxiety that the patient feels compelled to seek professional opinions and/or help.
3. *Threshold of inconvenience*: The condition interferes with valued behaviors or activities.

All of these are relative and variable. Discomfort can be immediate, intense, and unbearable, or it can become unbearable after hours or days have passed. "Why didn't you come right after you fell down?" inquires the doctor, rather exasperated. "It didn't hurt so much then," replies the patient, "and I could move it, so I figured it was only a sprain, not a break." Here, low initial pain, interpreted through a specific EM (e.g., "if it don't hurt, then it ain't broke") kept the patient from coming to the ED in a timely manner. The doctor's exasperation, however, is surely communicated to the patient, who is made to feel he has done something wrong.

Anxiety is in the eye of the anxious one. For many people, vomiting or urinating bright, red blood would likely create sufficient anxiety to spur a quick trip to the ED. A deep, nasty gash could trigger the same. But anything could trigger anxiety. The mother bringing her baby in at 2:00 p.m. because the child did not eat lunch has reached her own anxiety threshold. So, too, had the man who was finally frightened enough after 36 hours of mild but constant chest pain. From the staff perspective, the woman should not have become anxious because her baby had not eaten lunch. The fellow with the chest pain should have become anxious a whole lot sooner. Yet to him, not the pain but its persistence triggered the decision to seek emergency treatment. In both cases, staff feel frustration, and this frustration can be perceived by patients. Staff believe that their job is to treat "real" sicknesses or accidents, and to do so in a timely manner. Patients are often perceived as thwarting these efforts.

Inconvenience is typically viewed as an illegitimate justification for postponing treatment or for coming to the ED in the first place. A woman comes in with an ankle sprain that occurred three or four days earlier. She has four children who must be driven to school daily. She participates in a rotating carpool with friends and neighbors. The sprain now prevents her from stepping on the brake pedal with force, and she fears this will prevent her from fulfilling her driving obligations for the other carpool parents. A young man comes in with a three-day-old problem because tomorrow he must leave for reserve army duty. A young woman comes in with a cough she has had for days. She comes in now because she leaves on a vacation at 6:00 a.m. She has a regular physician, but his office will not open until 9:00 a.m.

Almost all ED visits reflect some social, economic, or other nonmedical component. An elderly woman drags her husband into the ED to have his heart examined. She claims that he has been acting strangely lately, been out of breath, and may be having a heart attack. He denies feeling sick. She has demanded that he come to the ED to "settle this once and for all!" It is a power struggle as much as it is a medical event.

A middle-aged man brings his boss into the ED. He has insisted the boss accompany him to prove to his boss that he really is sick and really should be excused from work (with sick pay, of course). The motive for the visit is economic as well as medical.

When patients such as these come to the ED for proof of sickness, staff may become frustrated. This is not a proper reason for seeking emergency care and tying up the time of busy professionals. Resentment of patients can be a result.

THE DOUBLE BIND

In all of these instances, staff feel beleaguered by patients who should not have come in the first place or who should have come at a more appropriate time. To many ED staff, patients should know what is appropriate to bring to the ED for treatment and when it is appropriate to bring it. Of course, once in the ED, patients should shut up and offer concise information only—not opinions, diagnoses, or treatment suggestions of their own. In this way, patients are put in a double bind, an uncomfortable situation in which they are punished for (on the one hand) not knowing medicine and (on the other hand) for audaciously claiming to know some medicine by requesting specific treatment.

"Why didn't you come in earlier?" exclaims the nurse to a 40-year-old white professional-looking male who presents around midnight with a deep, encrusted gash over his eye. The cut had occurred early that same morning.

"I had a lot to do, and it stopped bleeding, so I figured it could wait until I had time," the patient explains. "I came in for some stitches. Can you minimize the scarring?"

The nurse is frustrated by this patient, and testily replies: "No, we can't just sew it up like that and make it look nice! It's dried completely open. Now it has to be cleaned out, which won't be fun, and you'll probably have a much more obvious scar than if you'd come in sooner!"

Here, the nurse verbally punishes the patient for both presenting at the wrong time and daring to suggest the course of treatment.

A 35-year-old, middle-class white woman presents with a sore throat. "I'm leaving on vacation tomorrow," she adds, "and I know exactly what I need to get rid of it." She tells the triage nurse that she has had this same kind of sore throat before, and that a specific, named antibiotic always cures it quickly. She simply wants a prescription. She is assigned to a treatment cubicle and waits. Another nurse comes in to take a preliminary history and is given the same request. The frustrated patient waits even longer until a physician comes in. She reiterates her familiarity with the type of sore throat (e.g., "I've had this half a dozen times before") and requests the specific antibiotic. "This antibiotic always hits the sore throat fast. I've got to leave tomorrow morning, and I need this now to knock it out so I can enjoy the vacation."

The physician demurs, tells her he is calling for lab tests consisting of a throat culture and a blood analysis. Upon hearing of the blood test, the woman is now even more frustrated. The physician informs her that she may be suffering from anemia. The woman is furious over the fact that the physician has not taken her sore throat ideas seriously, and has further inserted a totally unexpected EM (anemia) into the interaction. She ultimately gets a prescription for the very antibiotic she wants but leaves extremely dissatisfied with the ED.

"She thinks she's the doctor," comments the physician, "and then she demands special treatment just because she's going on vacation to enjoy herself tomorrow." During the entire interaction, the doctor was coolly professional.

Harried ED staff may overlook the fact that the patient has a *life* in addition to a cough, pain, or gash. In Chapter 4, we discussed the importance of the various roles that define each person's life and identity. These roles are brought to the ED, just as they are brought to the physician's office or hospital bed. Even before patients come to the ED, their various roles and identities interact with the physical problem to enhance or retard time-appropriate, health-seeking behavior. It is precisely because these roles define our lives that we seek treatment when we are sick. We want to resume the roles, identities, and activities disrupted by the problem. All patients bring their threatened identities with them to the ED. Thus, staff must be sensitive to patients' reasons for coming in *now*. The question "Why didn't you come in sooner?" is essentially irrelevant. Knowing what is *presently* bothering the patient enough to trigger an ED visit can help staff establish quick rapport and design a treatment regimen that is more likely to be followed. The woman leaving for vacation tomorrow morning will likely not follow a recommendation of several days' bed rest. Moreover, her travels may make it difficult or inconvenient for her to take medication three or four times daily. Here, a once-a-day medication will more likely result in compliance.

TAKING PATIENTS SERIOUSLY

This is what it boils down to, really: for whatever reason, patients have decided to define their problem as an emergency and bring it to your hospital. In a number of ways, staff can demonstrate that they do—or do not—take these patients seriously. Patients want to be greeted by someone who knows enough emergency medicine to appreciate their problem. Patients want to be admitted to the treatment area quickly. They may not want to be shunted aside to an obvious urgent care or fast-track area that effectively tells them their claim to be an emergency patient is not taken seriously by staff.

Not that a fast-track facility in the ED automatically generates lower satisfaction; perhaps it just should not be too obviously identifiable. Fast track could be a separate process rather than a clearly separate place.

Patients come to the ED loaded with all of the cultural baggage we discussed in Chapter 4. They have sifted through symptoms and decided which were relevant. They have sifted through their own and their friends' and family's explanations about what they have and what should be done (their EM). To a lesser or greater degree, the problem affects them emotionally. To some extent, it has disrupted or threatened important roles and identities. The problem may also have shunted them into a sick role that they have successfully acted out at home and will act out in the ED. All of this is brought with the physical problem. Staff responses to these issues affect the patient's evaluation of care.

A sixty-year-old white male presents with his wife, complaining about a swollen, sore foot. He repeatedly asks the nurse, and subsequently the physician, whether he should be prescribed a footbath—something like Epsom salts—in which to soak his swollen foot. The physician ignores the request, explaining that the man's problem is internal, not external. An antibiotic is prescribed and the physician leaves. The patient and wife are both vocally upset. To them, an external problem, such as a swollen foot, should be treated with an external solution.

Note that the couple do not view the swelling as a symptom; rather, it is the problem. Their EM results in dissatisfaction when the physician ignores their very clear concerns. He did not take them seriously, and they knew it.

MORAL EVALUATIONS OF PATIENTS

In a seminal study of ED staff attitudes toward patients, Roth and Douglas (1983) note that staff have a pretty clear idea of who is an appropriate patient. Good patients present at the proper time with problems that are truly emergent. They are grateful for treatment. They cooperate. They answer questions concisely and produce relevant information. They are not demanding or complaining. They tolerate discomfort "like adults" and try not to make noise that could upset other patients. They do not pretend to know as much medicine as the doctors. Ideally, in fact, they know nothing but their symptoms, which are presented clearly and accurately. They do not conjecture about causes or cures. Friends and relatives who accompany good patients comport themselves with calm, dignity, appreciation, and understanding about delays and treatment protocols.

In addition, good patients present with proper problems. Not only are they emergent, but they are ideally not the patient's fault (Becker et al. 1961, 322). Nor are their medical problems caused by disreputable activities (e.g., fights, unsafe sex, dangerous acts such as motorcycling or in-line skating). A good patient does not acquire the problem or present to the emergency staff while under the influence of alcohol or drugs. A good patient pays for care in one way or another and is not a freeloader.

Patients share many values with medical staff. They themselves may find their problems embarrassing or deserving of disdain.

> An 80-year-old man presents at the ED complaining that he lost consciousness and fell on the sidewalk. He banged his head and wants it attended to. The physician suspects the patient may have suffered a stroke and orders appropriate tests. The old man converses with a volunteer, confiding that he really did not lose consciousness until *after* he fell. Rather shamefacedly, he admits that he fell while attempting to kick a can that was lying on the sidewalk. "It was a childish thing to do," he says. He did not tell the doctor because he felt ashamed to be so "stupid." Here, the patient brings his dignity with him to the ED, and it results in a lie to the physician.

The point is that patients—anticipating (deservedly or not) disdain or ridicule—may lie to staff or attempt to mislead them. Given the brief one-shot nature of the emergency encounter, accurate histories must be elicited and cooperation encouraged. Thus, staff attitudes toward patients must support the goals of emergency treatment. This is accomplished when staff attitudes are observably caring, supportive, and sympathetic. By "observably," I mean that tone of voice, body language, and actions demonstrate a clear, caring attitude.

Professional ED staff are largely middle class or above. Like patients, staff cannot leave their roles, identities, values, and prejudices at home. Drunks are disliked and treated coldly. Frequent flyers are the butts of jokes and made to wait. Fifteen-year-old single mothers are viewed with distaste, as well as with sorrow or disgust. Medicaid patients are often perceived as freeloaders and disdained. I have heard Medicaid patients referred to by staff as "gold-carders"—a judgmental reference to the fact that these patients can get good care without having to pay. I have also heard ED physicians talk of a "brown alert" (referring to feces) when a particularly high number of Medicaid patients were present. Of course, this probably does not happen in your ED, but it happens in some. For whatever reason, it is not unusual for Medicaid patients to spend more time waiting than do privately insured patients.

I have come across all of these as causes for staff resentment of various types of patients. We are not talking about all emergency staff, or even most of them. But all staff are human and cannot avoid frustration with some patients at some time. These frustrations can affect staff judgments of the legitimacy of patient claims to emergency status and proper emergency treatment. Treatment will indeed be given, but the patient (customer) may pay a price.

Roth and Douglas (1983) find that staff may attempt to punish patients who offend their sense of moral propriety or offend their professional status by presenting with unworthy problems. Punishment takes various forms. Patients may be made to wait or may not be looked in on by nurses. Interaction may be cool and professional but not friendly or comforting, or patients may be labeled.

LABELING

Verbal labels may be generic or patient specific. The disheveled guy with the torn shirt that looks like a cape may be referred to as "Superman." The young man whimpering as his knife-fight wound is stitched may be denigrated as "Mr. Macho." More generically, the woman with vague stomach symptoms but no test-revealed pathology may be a "crock." The guy who has been to the ED three times in the past four weeks is a "frequent flyer." I came across an ED where drunks, druggies, and patients with vague, untreatable symptoms were referred to as "oids" (as in "humanoids"). Most "oids" were Medicaid patients. In yet another ED, staff would refer to similar patients as "3-footers," "4-footers," or "5-footers" (referring to turkey wing span). A "5-footer" was a real turkey.

Patients' moral legitimacy, as well as their legitimacy as ED patients, may also be judged and labeled by staff. The 14-year-old girl presenting with low stomach pains may be referred to as a "crotch case" and assumed to be suffering from a sexually transmitted disease. I saw one such young woman being asked if she were taking any medication. She responded by saying that she was taking birth control pills. Staff asked for the pill dispenser and taped it to her chart, which was hung on the chart board in full view of everyone on both sides of the counter. An acquaintance of mine reports:

> I was in the emergency room for something, and I was waiting to see the doctor. I could hear him talking to a patient in the bed next to me on the other side of the curtain. She was a young black girl, about 14 or so, and had come in complaining about stomach pains. Her mother was with her. The doctor asks the girl, "Are you sexually active?"
>
> Can you believe that? Right in front of her mother, he asks her that! How embarrassing for the girl!

Here, the physician may be responding to what he believes to be immoral behavior by confronting (punishing) the girl about her sexuality directly in front of her mother. The physician also may have been reflecting his personal stereotypes about blacks and their sexual behavior. The net result, however, is that a moral judgment was made and the patient punished. As a side issue, these comments were overheard by another patient, who was also turned off by the interaction. Walls are thin in EDs. I have seen nurses stand just outside the curtain to purposely and loudly discuss a mother's (in)ability to care for her child, who was in for ingesting some household cleaner kept under the sink. Their comments were designed to punish.

Labeling need not be verbal. Patients who are viewed as behavioral problems or disdained for one reason or another may be assigned to "Room 11." Every ED has a "Room 11," which is usually at a distance from the nursing station and to which are assigned sensitive patients such as rape victims or, more usually, disreputable or unruly patients, or teenage girls with vague stomach pains or obvious STDs. Even if placed in a standard treatment room, a disdained patient may receive minimal visits from nurses and cool interaction from physicians. Recall Chapter 4's discussion about the effect of labeling on staff interaction with patients.

DELAYS AND WAITING TIME

In the past few years, there have been dozens of conferences on reducing ED delays. What, however, is a delay? Do we count total time spent in the ED, or only time spent in a waiting room outside the treatment area? Or time spent waiting in a treatment cubicle? And are we talking about real time or perceived time?

People talk about getting patients in and out in less than 30 minutes. Is this realistic? Is it even desirable? Dr. Jim Espinosa, head of the ED of Overlook Hospital in Summit, New Jersey, reports that ED satisfaction scores rose as total time decreased—that is, until patients began spending an average of less than 30 minutes in the ED. At that point, satisfaction scores started falling again. Espinosa believes the decline was because patients began to feel that their examination and treatment was rushed and not thorough.

By and large, the longer that patients are in the ED, the less satisfied they are with overall care (see Figure 11.1). After the first hour, satisfaction drops by 3 to 5 points per hour. Patients who have to stay over four hours are typically sicker, require more observation and treatment, and appear to tolerate the additional time. This suggests that if you want to reduce total ED time and improve satisfaction, then focus on getting the less acute patients out faster.

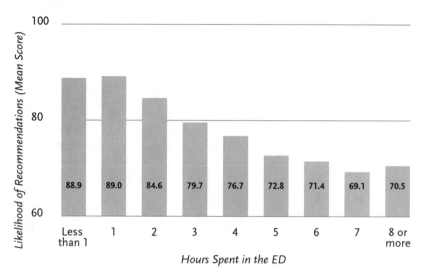

Figure 11.1. Likelihood of Recommending the ED by Hours Spent in the ED

Note: n = 1,409,503 patients, 1,354 facilities.
Source: Press Ganey Associates. 2005.

How much of the total time spent in the ED constitutes a delay? And what is a delay?

Consider the following typical patient experience:

1. Arrival.
2. Interview with admitting personnel.
3. Triage (if triage nurse is not doing the admitting).
4. Possible wait in external waiting room if ED is busy.
5. Admission to treatment area.
6. Nurse takes vitals and information.
7. Physician visits—may treat or call for tests.
8. Technologist or nurse takes blood, EKG, etc.
9. Possible trip to x-ray.
10. X-ray taken.
11. Wait for escort back to ED treatment room.

12. Physician returns with results. Discusses. Explains, treats, or prescribes.
13. Nurse "closes." Discharge or slated for admission to inpatient bed.
14. Wait for transport upstairs, if necessary.

This sequence is pretty typical and logical, but not for the patient. The patient cannot predict these events. Between each event is a potential delay while the patient waits for an unknown someone to do an unknown something. The typical patient experiences at least 8 or 9 of these events and as many as all 14. There may be at least two waits for the doctor.

Most patients spend little or no time in the lobby waiting area; almost all the time is spent back in the treatment area. Patients view the entire time in the treatment area as treatment time. Treatment is not over until they leave the ED, so until they are discharged, they are theoretically waiting to be treated.

Because the physician is the key person who diagnoses, treats, and releases them, patients equate total time in the ED with time spent waiting for the physician to treat them.

Figure 11.2 illustrates total time spent in the ED and its effect on patients' judgments of the appropriateness of the time spent waiting for the physician. Given our previous discussion, we view the wait for the physician as equivalent to the patient's judgment of the appropriateness of the total time spent in the treatment area. Clearly, because most of the patient's time is spent in the treatment area, the less time spent there, the more the patient views this time as appropriate.

It is important to note that those patients who are very satisfied with the time spent in the treatment area are still spending an average of three hours in the ED; therefore, reducing time is not in itself the key to satisfaction with emergency care. The best method of gauging the effect of delays on patients is via satisfaction surveys, not time logs by staff.

Figure 11.2. Effect of Total Hours Spent in the ED on Patient Judgments of Appropriateness of Waiting Time to See the Doctor

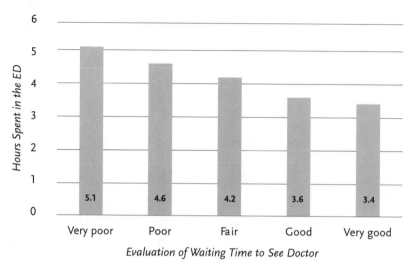

Evaluation of Waiting Time to See Doctor

Note: n = 1,409,503 patients, 1,354 facilities.
Source: Press Ganey Associates. 2004.

We must be very careful to distinguish between total actual time spent in the ED and patients' judgments of the *appropriateness* of this time. The correlations in Figure 11.3 on the following page are most revealing: Patient satisfaction with the overall ED experience is definitely affected by judgments of the appropriateness of time spent in the waiting room and in the treatment area. Correlations of .592 and .648 are quite high. Not surprisingly, patients view time in the treatment area as somewhat more important than time in the external waiting room. Far more interesting, however, is the correlation of how well the patient was informed about delays with overall satisfaction. A correlation of .732 is very high. What it tells us is that when patients are given information about what to expect, when to expect it, and why it did not happen when expected, they are far more satisfied with the overall ED experience.

Figure 11.3. Likelihood of Recommending ED

Likelihood Correlated with:	Actual Waiting Time	Waiting Room Wait	Treatment Wait	Informed About Delays
	–.160	.592	.648	.732

Note: All correlations are significant at the .000 level.

The importance of explaining events and delays is strikingly exhibited in the rather formidable graph in Figure 11.4.

We have already looked at the relationship between total time in the ED and patient judgments of the appropriateness of the wait to see the physician. The longer the total time, the lower the satisfaction with the wait. But what if patients are given explanations about what is happening and why it is taking so long?

The darkest bars reflect very poor information about delays—and very low satisfaction with the wait to be treated by the doctor. Note that satisfaction with the wait for a physician drops about 13 points—from a peak of 37 on a 100-point scale—as the hours pass. The lightest bars are quite different. They reflect very good information about delays. Note that for the same total time spent, patients rate the wait to be treated 60 to 70 points higher when good explanations are given. Moreover, with the good explanations, there is virtually no drop in satisfaction as the hours pass! What this shows, again, is that information and perception of *appropriateness* of time underlie satisfaction, not actual hours spent in the ED. *The more information given about what is happening, the more that patients view the passing time as acceptable.*

You will notice that of the patients receiving very poor information (i.e., none), those in the ED for less than an hour are still quite dissatisfied with care. This could reflect Jim Espinosa's conclusion that patients who are discharged after a very short period of time may be inclined to feel that their health issue was not taken seriously.

Figure 11.4. Patient's Likelihood to Recommend by Wait Time and Information Received About Delays

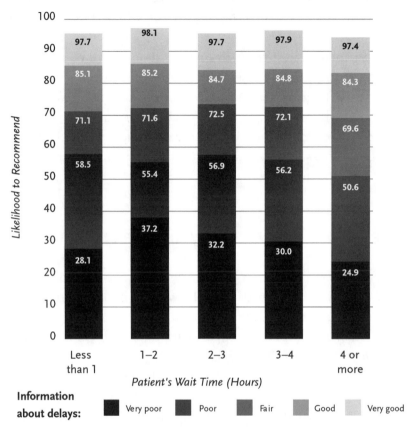

Note: n = 1,409,503 patients, 1,354 hospitals; Jan. 1–Dec. 31, 2004.
Source: Press Ganey Associates. 2005.

Resetting the Clock

One of our client EDs noted low scores for waiting time. They solved the problem simply. Anyone who has contact with the patient —from admitting clerk to nurse to doctor to lab tech to whoever— is responsible for telling the patient what will happen next, who will do it, and approximately when it will happen. Overestimating the time until the next event is preferable to underestimating it. Whenever the doctor or nurse enters the treatment cubicle, they apologize for any delay. The results have been remarkable. Satisfaction with overall care has escalated, as has satisfaction with the time spent in the treatment area.

The patient's clock starts ticking the moment he or she is admitted, and it keeps on ticking throughout the whole treatment. However, if patients are given new information about when the next event will occur (e.g., "It'll take about 20 minutes for me to analyze this blood and for the doctor to get back to you"), then they reset their clocks for that time. Otherwise, the only referent is the entire time spent from the moment of admission.

THE IDEAL EMERGENCY DEPARTMENT

More than anything, simply knowing what is important to patients offers a solution to the question of "How do we improve satisfaction with our ED?" Figure 11.5 presents a list correlating all items in the Press Ganey ED satisfaction survey with the likelihood of patients recommending the ED to others.

All items on the survey are significantly linked to satisfaction; however, those near the top of the list (i.e., those with higher correlation coefficients) have a closer relationship to the likelihood of recommending. By focusing attention on these issues, EDs can make significant improvements. Note that the majority of key items are interaction related. By far, the most important issue is the degree to which staff care about the patient as a person. Clearly, during the brief, anxiety-charged emergency experience, patients expect more than technical competence. In their study of ED patient satisfaction, Hall and Press (1996, 527) conclude,

> Large numbers—typically the majority—of emergency patients present with fairly simple problems (not necessarily to them, of course!). As they receive appropriately simple technical care (if any) and leave

Figure 11.5. Issues Correlated with Likelihood of Recommending ED

	Correlation Coefficient
Degree to which staff cared about you as person	0.79
How well you were kept informed about delays you may have experienced in the emergency room	0.72
How well your pain was controlled	0.72
Nurse's concern to keep you informed about your treatments	0.69
Staff concern to keep family or friends informed about your status during your course of treatment	0.69
Nurse's attention to your needs	0.69
Courtesy with which family or friends were treated	0.68
Doctor's concern for your comfort while treating you	0.68
Doctor's concern to keep you informed about your treatment	0.67
Information you were given about caring for yourself at home	0.67
Degree to which nurses took the time to listen to you	0.67
Waiting time in the treatment area, before you were seen by a doctor	0.67
Degree to which the doctor took the time to listen to you	0.66
Courtesy of the nurses	0.64
Courtesy of the doctor	0.64
Nurse's concern for your privacy	0.62
Waiting time before you were brought to the treatment area	0.62
Staff concern to let a family member or friend be with you while you were being treated	0.59
Helpfulness of the person who first asked you about your condition	0.58
Comfort of the waiting area	0.57
Waiting time before staff noticed your arrival	0.53
Concern shown for your comfort when your blood was drawn	0.52
Courtesy of person who took your blood	0.51
Waiting time for radiology test	0.51
Ease of giving your personal/insurance information	0.51
Privacy you felt when asked about your personal/insurance information	0.51
Courtesy of the person who took your personal/insurance information	0.50
Concern shown for your comfort during your test	0.47
Courtesy of the radiology staff	0.46

Note: n = 1,415,425 patients, 1,354 facilities; $p < 0.001$; Jan. 1–Dec. 31, 2004.
Source: Press Ganey Associates. 2005.

stabilized rather than cured, it is not surprising that various studies (as well as ours) conclude that interpersonal factors may contribute most to satisfaction with the ED.

Care in the ideal ED addresses these factors directly or indirectly. Following are general characteristics of an ideal ED—one in which concern for patient satisfaction drives all aspects of care, from physical plant to organization and interaction. We are not going to mention one obvious ideal—that the ED is big enough, modern enough, designed well enough, and staffed well enough to make a positive impression on patients regardless of any organizational or behavioral characteristics. In truth, you do not need a modern facility to satisfy anxious, uncomfortable patients who want attention, empathy, reassurance, and appropriate treatment. Modern, cheerful facilities help reduce patient anxiety, but to increase patient satisfaction significantly, far more is needed.

1. *First and foremost, the ideal ED is self-aware.* Its staff recognize that departmental organization is cultural in nature and is riddled with ritual and justifications, such as "We've always done it this way." The ideal ED approaches every rule, work habit, and protocol (that is not specifically mandated by law or regulatory agencies) from a perspective of zero-based budgeting. That is, each action must be justified by more than an appeal to tradition. In most EDs, for example, nursing notes are typically written out in narrative form. For most patient problems, however, a simple checklist format might work well. This reduces time spent documenting common presenting symptoms, health history, and so forth.

Union Hospital in Union, New Jersey, demonstrated zero-based budgeting when it redesigned its triage process. Standing orders were written for many common ailments such as abdominal pain, ankle injuries, and others. The triage nurse can initiate a set of standing x-ray protocols, order a CBC or other routine blood work, and initiate an IV. Thus, patients perceive that they are being taken seriously and much time is also saved. In this case, it was decided that many routine aspects of diagnosis or treatment did not demand a physician's time.

Jim Espinosa recognized that EDs were ritually set up to focus more on admitted than discharged patients, who are typically in the majority. In an effort to satisfy the bulk of their customers, waiting time was cut in half (Espinosa and Kosnik 1998). One of the things they did was to examine the need to have all x-rays assessed by a radiology specialist prior to delivery of the film to the emergency physician. They decided that this was a time-consuming ritual that could be abolished. Films were already delivered directly to the ED doctors during evenings and weekends. According to literature research, emergency physicians had been determined to be quite capable of accurately recognizing whether a problem was visible in the x-ray. Overlook Hospital subsequently standardized this practice for all shifts.

Lourdes Hospital in Binghamton, New York, uses the same procedure, but also has a radiologist look at all films within two hours and report back to the ED physician if there is any difference in interpretation.

2. *The ideal ED has some provision for fast-track treatment that appears to the patient to be part of the ordinary ED process.* Thus, many non-acute patients can be seen more quickly without being made to feel that their problem is not taken seriously. Fast-track areas could be staffed with registered nurses (RNs) and physician assistants (PAs), but patients will likely be more satisfied if a doctor makes even a brief appearance.

3. *Everyone in the ideal ED thinks entrepreneurially.* All staff recognize that patients are also customers and have economic value to the broader medical center network. To legitimize this orientation, both the CEO and CFO have led workshops attended by all ED staff, especially physicians, informing them of the economic importance to the entire institution of an entrepreneurially oriented ED. In addition, attendance at a customer service workshop is mandated—again, this mandate includes physicians.

4. *Everyone, from receptionists to physicians, knows the ED's latest satisfaction scores.* Patient satisfaction is a permanent agenda item at department meetings, and physicians are required to attend.

5. *If the emergency physicians belong to a practice management group, then their contract with the hospital puts the group at risk for some compensation reduction if patient satisfaction scores fall below a target number.* At the same time, the hospital is committed to providing additional compensation if satisfaction levels exceed the target.

6. *Group discussions are organized and managed by a facilitator who can lead staff to confront their feelings about who is or is not a "legitimate" emergency patient.* Discussion deals with issues of moral evaluation as well as medical evaluation of "deserving" patients. Discussion also confronts the potential effect of staff attitudes on their interaction with and management of patients. Staff may also need to confront elements of racism and other socioeconomic prejudices that can affect labeling of and interaction with patients.

7. *The admitting desk is situated in such a manner as to maximize the potential for privacy.*

8. *Admitting personnel are empathetic, knowledgeable, and mature in both manner and appearance (particularly if not an RN), thus fostering trust in his or her ability to understand the problem and take it seriously.* Many people are uncomfortable or embarrassed telling very personal things to someone who looks relatively young and/or who does not appear to be a nurse or physician. Ideally, the admitting person is the triage nurse.

9. *Bedside registration is the rule.* The patient is ushered into the treatment area before financial or other registration information is elicited. This says, "Your problem is taken more seriously than your insurance status."

10. *Patients cannot see into one another's rooms.* They are asked if they want their door or curtain closed or left open (so they can see the staff and be distracted by the action).

11. *Every person who contacts the patient explains what is going to happen next, who will do it, and when it will occur.* Every person

who subsequently interacts with the patient does the same. Staff who have been delayed apologize to the patient.

12. *The patient is offered a blanket, pillow, or other comfort-maker.* If appropriate, a soft drink or water and/or snack is offered.

13. *A chair or two are available in the treatment cubicle for visitors.* And there is a stool for the doctor to sit on, a local phone, and a TV. A soft drink and snack machine are conveniently located out in the waiting room; these take tokens that are provided at no cost by the admitting desk.

14. *A nurse looks in on the patient frequently, asking if everything's ok—and sounds like she sincerely wants to know.*

15. *Friends and relatives who accompany the patient are treated in a friendly, courteous manner.* Staff demeanor communicates to guests that their presence is expected and welcomed, not merely tolerated.

16. *If the ED is a busy one, then volunteer patient liaisons make the round of patients.* These liaisons should keep the patients company, chat, perform small errands, explain ED routine or culture (e.g., why the delay, why the doctor has not come back yet, why the patient in the next cubicle is being treated sooner even though he was admitted later, etc.).[1]

17. *The physician introduces himself or herself and sits so as to minimize intimidation.* The physician touches the patient and chats for a second of two before getting down to business.

18. *The physician elicits the patient's EM.* Given the shortness of time, all that is required are two questions: "What do you think is the matter?" (this can be omitted for a number of obvious injuries), and "What do you think should be done?" Many patients will not respond or will say, "I don't know—you're the doctor." This happens a lot, but you have to ask. If patients respond, then their EM is at least listened to and, where appropriate, accommodated. This encourages trust and empathy. It shows that the patient is taken seriously.

19. *The patient is asked why he or she is coming in now if the problem occurred significantly earlier.* If at all possible, treatment protocols should reflect the patient's present need (e.g., social,

recreational, emotional) for treatment. After telling patients how to care for themselves at home, physicians elicit some information about the patient's ability to comply with discharge instructions. Care regimens are adjusted accordingly. If post-ED care regimens conflict with accustomed living habits or special occasions, then the result will often (if not usually) be noncompliance.

20. *Patients are not placed in a double-bind situation.* Staff do not expect them to know when it is appropriate to come in or what problems are appropriate for emergency treatment.

21. *Patients' emotions are expected and tolerated as long as they do not disrupt the ED or significantly affect other patients.* Staff assume that patients may be suffering, scared, threatened, and embarrassed. This is an ED, not a bank lobby.

22. *Professional and social prejudices are hidden from patients.* Sexually active teens, overly worried mothers, frequent flyers, and overly demanding Medicaid patients have not come to the ED to be morally corrected or punished.

23. *Staff never discuss patients where they can be overheard.*

24. *Everyone (i.e., doctors, nurses, lab techs, and therapists) explains what he or she is doing and why.*

25. *Closing is done by the physician, not a nurse.* Ideally, the doctor sits during the final statement and instructions. Usually, this is the time for asking if the patient has any questions. If the doctor's voice and body language say "I'm on my way out of here, make it fast," then it is unlikely that the patient will ask anything. Such behavior also encourages noncompliance.

26. *Patients are phoned later in the evening after discharge by a nurse who asks how they are doing, if they have any questions, and if they have followed through on the discharge instructions.* Union Hospital in Union, New Jersey, does this, and the call is scripted to make it easier and faster. Very busy EDs may not be able to do this. Lourdes Hospital in Binghamton, New York, does not phone everyone, just those whose diagnoses represent conditions judged to create a risk for the patient. Patients with these diagnoses are

phoned the next day. Patients who leave against medical advice (AMA) are also phoned.

These are but a few characteristics of the ideal ED. The list could be much longer. Note that almost all elements require modest behavioral or attitudinal changes rather than construction or major reorganization of tasks. Establishment of a fast-track service might be an exception, but even this could be managed with imaginative staffing changes using existing facilities. Every ED in the country already exhibits many of these ideal characteristics.

CONCLUSIONS

In two senses, the ED is the gateway to the hospital. On the one hand, many patients are admitted to the inpatient sector from the ED. The ED experience can predispose the patient positively or negatively to events and interactions that follow. On the other hand, for thousands of prospective customers of the hospital and its associated services, the ED may be the initial marketing experience.

Most important, of course, is that for all who enter the ED, care must be provided in such as way as to maximize its effectiveness. Because the contact between emergency patient and staff is brief, intense, and to some extent unavoidably impersonal, special care must be taken in designing protocols for patient/staff interaction and for controlling the patient's experience in the facility. Attention to patient satisfaction can have a significant effect on patient management and outcome in this unique, intense, stress-laden context.

ACTION FOR SATISFACTION

1. Approach every rule, work habit, and protocol from the perspective of zero-based budgeting.
2. Create a fast-track treatment that will not be noticeably different to the patient.

3. Think (and encourage staff to think) like an entrepreneur.
4. Post satisfaction scores.
5. Hold physicians accountable for satisfaction scores.
6. Conduct discussions about staff attitudes in interactions with and management of patients.
7. Position the admitting desk to maximize patient privacy and hire an RN to man the desk.
8. Implement bedside registration.
9. Provide privacy for each patient. Staff never discuss patients where they can be overheard.
10. Make it a part of standard procedure to communicate with patients about what will happen next, who will do it, and when it will occur.
11. Provide for the patient's comfort with extra pillows, blankets, snacks, chairs for visitors, phones, and so forth.
12. Make it possible for nurses to check in on patients frequently. Teach staff to respond to patients and their visitors in a friendly, sincere manner.
13. Create a patient liaison position to care for the non-clinical needs of patients.
14. Train physicians to increase patient satisfaction by sitting when in the patient's presence, chatting with the patient, eliciting and listening to the patient's EM, and so forth.
15. Train staff to listen to the patient's reasoning for seeking treatment, respect patient's knowledge levels and emotional responses to illness, and hide prejudices.
16. Make it standard procedure that a patient's final instructions are given by a physician who allows time for questions.
17. Phone patients after care to follow up on discharge instructions and provide further explanation if necessary.

NOTE

1. Obviously, the patient has to give consent for this, but most are more than happy to have someone to chat with. Obviously, too, staffing is the major issue. You would

want the liaisons during the busiest times—especially the 4:00 p.m. to midnight shift. Liaisons can be standard volunteers or employees. Here is another idea: I started programs in two local EDs in South Bend over 20 years ago, and they are still running strong. Contact the social science departments at a local college or university (e.g., anthropology, sociology, psychology, economics; also try philosophy and theology). Ask if anyone is teaching a course having to do with healthcare (e.g., medical anthropology, medical economics, medical ethics). The professor will jump at the chance to have students get first-hand experience in a local ED. Offer to host a lab or practicum for students in the course.

Each student will take a four-hour shift in your ED once a week. Ideally, you will have all seven days covered from 4:00 p.m. to midnight. (It is easier than you think to get students to choose the weekend shifts—they are busier and more exciting.) The students get real-life ED experience, plus great material for term papers. You get free liaisons (limit the program to juniors and seniors only) who are well-educated, responsible, articulate, and kept in line by their professor, who can affect their grades if they do not show up for a shift or who break your behavioral rules (see Press and Smith 1986).

REFERENCES

Becker, H. S., B. Geer, E. C. Hughes, and A. L. Strauss. 1961. *Boys in White: Student Culture in Medical School*. Chicago: University of Chicago Press.

Espinosa, J., and L. Kosnik. 1998. "The Overlook Hospital Emergency Department's Journey to Align with the Voices of Its Customers." Press Ganey Success Story contest entry, November.

Hall, M., and I. Press. 1996. "Keys to Patient Satisfaction in the Emergency Department: Results of a Multiple Facility Study." *Hospital and Health Services Administration* 41 (4): 515–32.

Mayer, T., and R. Cates. 2004. *Leadership for Great Customer Service*. Chicago: Health Administration Press.

McCaig, L. F. 1994. "National Hospital Ambulatory Medical Care Survey: 1992 Emergency Department Summary." Press release, March 2. Washington, DC: NCHS (HHS).

Press, I., and D. Smith. 1986. "Premedical Students as Patient and Family Liaisons in the Emergency Department: A Strategy for Patient Satisfaction." *Journal of Emergency Nursing* 12 (1): 23–5.

Roth, J. A., and D. J. Douglas. 1983. *No Appointment Necessary: The Hospital Emergency Department in the Medical Services World*. New York: Irvington Publishers, Inc.

CHAPTER 12

Implementing Change

AN INSTITUTIONWIDE PATIENT satisfaction focus will be more successful than a piecemeal attempt to improve satisfaction. With the broad approach, everyone is brought on board at the same time, and pockets of resistance are minimized and readily identifiable. Beginning small or making piecemeal attempts at cultural change to test the waters indicates a lack of institutional confidence and commitment. This final chapter outlines the steps needed to implement an effective program.

GETTING STARTED

An official, broadly planned, institutionwide plan backed by universal training, discussion, monitoring (measurement), expectations, and rewards is also much easier than a piecemeal attempt. When everyone in the organization reflects and reinforces the values, individuals stay committed. Peer pressure alone will keep things moving. Such group pressures keep cultures going on a day-to-day basis. Resist the temptation to begin things small and "see how they work."

Establish a Context

Begin with a plan. Contact other hospitals to learn what they have done to make patient satisfaction a core element of their culture. Ask, "What has worked and what hasn't? How did you set goals? What rewards and incentives have you used? How did you handle staff who were reluctant to buy in? How did you involve your docs?"

Initiate a major kickoff campaign long before you start holding people accountable for patient satisfaction. First, generate internal publicity. Explain what is going to happen, describe the goals, and focus on the advantages for staff, physicians, and patients. Require each group to prepare a written report outlining what they see as their role in the satisfaction culture. You may want to create a campaign name, perhaps an acronym for various attributes you are stressing. For example, Holy Cross Hospital in Chicago, Illinois, named its campaign "SERVE": Service, Excellence, Respect for patients, Value, and Enthusiasm. You can easily invent something similar.

Memorial Hospital Pembroke in Pembroke Pines, Florida, groups its customer service behavioral standards under the following headings: professionalism, attitude, teamwork, effective communication, pride, and safety awareness. Each heading became an acronym for the specific standards. Acronyms can be useful as mnemonic devices that help staff remember specific points. For example, "attitude" is broken down into a behavioral standard for each letter of the word:

Attitude makes a difference. Be positive.
Thank each and every customer.
Treat each person as if he or she is the most important person in the organization.

Initiate a connection. Say hello.
Take them there. Escort lost customers.
Understand the customer's needs.
Display appropriate body language.
Exceed our customers' expectations.

Establish a Satisfaction Baseline

Before starting on a patient satisfaction initiative, you should begin measuring patient satisfaction. If you already have a survey going, then your QI teams can practice problem identification and problem solving with the most recent survey results. How will you handle communications with your lowest-scoring nursing unit or department? How can you prevent them from becoming overly defensive? How will you encourage them to improve? How will goals be established for future improvements?

Control the Metaphor

Management must stress that low satisfaction scores at the beginning of the process are a challenge and an opportunity—not a problem or occasion for punishment. The idea of linguistically converting "problems" into "opportunities" sounds a lot like spin-doctoring, but it works. What you call something is how you ultimately respond to it. By stressing that low scores are opportunities for improvement and recognition, staff come to view them as challenges and a chance to gather accolades and rewards. In this way, the satisfaction survey becomes a tool rather than a threat.

Leave No One Out!

If you are going to measure their performance, then staff have got to be involved from the beginning. Too often we hear of staff who have never seen their survey or data reports, or who did not participate in (or were allowed to bug-out of) initial orientation sessions about patient satisfaction and institutional expectations about performance. This is particularly the case with physicians.

Involve Your Doctors from the First

Ultimately, no satisfaction or quality improvement program can work if the physicians are not on board. Usually, they are the last to buy into the importance of patient satisfaction as a measure of the quality of care. Quite often, this lack of buy-in is caused by the physicians not being involved in the cultural change program from the beginning. Someone in management says, "The docs won't want this. You know how they are. Let's not involve them until it's working well." With this kind of attitude, the program likely *won't* work well. Physicians' influence (e.g., professional, moral, political) is too pervasive to be ignored. Your survey should contain some items about patient satisfaction with physicians. Make sure physicians are given the opportunity to at least comment on the survey items that involve their interaction with patients. Your chief of staff should be involved in discussions that identify potential causes and courses of action should scores, both in general and for individual physicians, be low. If you have a senior-level patient satisfaction committee, then a physician should definitely be on it.

Wabash Valley Practice Management, which manages a number of physician practices in hospitals around Terre Haute, Indiana, at first presented blind patient satisfaction scores to its physicians. No individual was identified, and no progress was made in satisfaction, either. Taking advantage of the competitive nature of physicians, they began identifying individual scores where all physicians could see them. Some physicians went into denial. For most of the physicians, however, the strategy worked, and satisfaction scores improved dramatically. Wabash Management points out that some of the busiest practices (i.e., highest patient-to-physician ratio) achieved highest patient satisfaction scores. This undermines the common excuse that "we have no time to spend on nonessential behaviors."

A note on involving physicians: The chief physician (e.g., chief of staff, chairman of the medical group, ED director) must be on board and must take responsibility for his or her staff's patient satisfaction effort, or it will not work. Only physicians have real credibility with other physicians. The physician leader must speak with low-scoring doctors, encouraging a search for possible causes and suggesting possible behavioral or practice changes. The survey manager for the hospital or practice (usually not a physician) should have previously spoken with the leader about possible causes that may be affecting the low-scoring physician's performance. If there are written survey comments, then the leader shares these with the physician. Patient satisfaction must always be an agenda item at medical staff meetings.

Try for Some Early Successes

Do not go for a single, long-term, "all or nothing" goal. Set goals of differing lengths, based on levels of difficulty. Start with a set of easily and quickly achievable score goals. You will generate stronger commitment if you continuously achieve successes along the way. Try to pick some low-hanging fruit. From your patient satisfaction data, select lower-scoring issues whose causes are pretty obvious and not too complex or expensive to address. Fix them. Celebrate the improvement in scores. Publicize it. Give out some rewards.

Prioritize Your Projects

To select targets for quality improvement, go beyond a priority index, which looks at scores plus the relationship of each item with overall satisfaction. Remember, lower scores and higher correlation with overall satisfaction means higher priority. Some issues may be of high priority yet are hard or expensive to implement. Target your projects by both priority and ease of implementation.

Memorial Medical Center in Johnstown, Pennsylvania, developed a useful nine-block grid for prioritizing improvement targets.

First, they looked at all of their patient survey questions and judged each issue on whether it would be easy, moderately easy, or difficult to improve. Then they created a priority index of all items on their satisfaction survey and split the list into even thirds, which they labeled high, medium, and low priority. Survey items were then apportioned into the appropriate box. They then did a final prioritization and gave each box a priority ranking as shown in Figure 12.1. The issues in box 1 were to be tackled first—easy-fix, low-hanging fruit with quick reinforcement), followed by issues in box 2, then box 3, and so forth. The higher the box number, the further in the future improvement was planned. Numbering the boxes is obviously a judgment call, and you might decide to order them differently. This kind of technique helps you to organize your improvement program with more hope of success. Do not pick projects ad hoc. When you rank order them with some logic and structure, the validity and utility of your survey data is reinforced. At the same time, it also reinforces the rationale (financial concerns as well as practicality) for your program's targets.

Forming Improvement Teams

Ideally, every employee in the hospital—from highest to lowest on the organizational chart—should be required to spend some time on a QI/patient satisfaction team or committee. No matter how modest the function of the team, when someone serves on it, he or she has a stake in furthering the overall mission.

Improvement teams can be formed upon various bases. Memorial Hospital Pembroke in Pembroke Pines, Florida, developed the following eight teams for its new program:

Figure 12.1. Project Prioritization Grid (with Survey Items Allocated to Each)

Relative Ease of Improving

	Easy	Moderately Easy	Difficult
High	**1** 18, 20, 29, 49	**2** 4, 5, 23, 26, 38, 42	**5** 10, 34, 35
Medium	**3** 2, 14, 30, 32, 33, 50	**4** 1, 3, 12, 43, 44	**6** 16, 37
Low	**7** 7, 8, 13, 21, 24, 45, 48	**8** 11, 28, 30, 40, 47	**9** 9, 15, 17, 19, 22, 25, 27, 39, 41, 46

Priority of Issue (vertical axis label)

Note: Based on a grid used by Memorial Medical Center, Johnstown, Pennsylvania.

1. Inpatient satisfaction
2. Outpatient satisfaction
3. Emergency satisfaction
4. Standards of behavior (for all in the hospital: scripting, etc.)
5. Reward and recognition
6. Service recovery
7. Physician satisfaction

8. Measurement (handling and disseminating the survey and data)

The inpatient satisfaction team, for example, was charged with improving the entire inpatient experience. One area they looked at was admission scores. They developed the following recommendations that were subsequently implemented:

1. Patients are greeted with a smile.
2. All patients are escorted to their area or units.
3. The welcome is scripted.
4. Delays are explained.
5. Waiting areas and lounges are to be renovated.
6. Coffee service is provided.
7. An admitting clerk visits each new patient the day after admission.
8. At this visit, clerk offers any personal care items patient may have forgotten.
9. Staff commit to very best performance at the outset.

Subsequent to their improvement program, overall patient satisfaction with Memorial improved dramatically.

You can create either situational teams to tackle ostensibly temporary problems or standing teams to work continually with ongoing issues. If you are undergoing significant construction, then a situational, "reducing construction irritants team" can work on tactics to reduce inconvenience to patients and to explain what is going on. If you have low scores for the admitting section of your survey, then a situational team can focus on it until the scores rise sufficiently. Many issues are relatively continuous. For example, there will always be complaints, and these could be investigated and remedial action recommended by a standing "complaint management team." Although you probably already have a service recovery program running and wide staff empowerment to deal with patient complaints, some group should keep track of complaints to identify patterns in the issues raised. A "reward and recognition team" could develop and manage hospitalwide rewards for satisfaction score improvement, exemplary service, and so forth.

All hospitalwide teams should consist of members from different departments. Of course, every department and unit should have its own standing patient satisfaction team, charged with monitoring survey results and organizing brainstorming sessions to deal with specific performance issues. All teams should have a percentage of their members rotate off each year, so as to maximize participation (and buy-in) by staff. The existence of specific departmental or unit teams does not preclude the necessity for some hospital-level teams to oversee and support them.

Baptist Health Care in Pensacola, Florida, created seven hospital-level support teams when they developed their patient satisfaction program. These teams include the following:

Measurement Team

Focus: To correctly measure and interpret progress.

Tasks:

1. Monitor weekly scores and publish results each Thursday. Results are announced in weekly department leader meeting and distributed by e-mail by Thursday afternoon.
2. Identify improvement opportunities.
3. Receive quarterly report from patient satisfaction measurement firm and assist departments in developing improvement plans.

Standards Team

Focus: To create behaviors that support the mission and values.

Tasks:

1. Develop Standards of Performance manual.
2. Coordinate "Standard of the Month" celebrations throughout hospital.
3. Develop policy that all job applicants must read and sign and agree to honor.

Communication Team

Focus: To develop mechanisms that give all employees access to information about the hospital and its policies.

Tasks:

1. Develop "communication boards" in each department.
2. Develop agenda for employee forums.

Linkage Team

Focus: To reward and recognize behaviors that align with the standards of performance.

Tasks:

1. Develop hospitalwide and department celebrations for achievements.
2. Develop "champions" program to recognize employees who go beyond.
3. Develop "legends" program to recognize employees who consistently go beyond.

Irritants Team

Focus: To identify and correct those behaviors, processes, and so forth that irritate our customers.

Tasks:

1. Review available data to determine irritants and develop improvement plans.
2. Initiate and develop service recovery program.

Physician Satisfaction Team

Focus: To build loyalty among physicians and to enhance patient satisfaction with physician services.

Tasks:

1. Create opportunities for dialog with physicians.
2. Include physicians in development of improvement strategies.
3. Measure physician satisfaction with the hospital.
4. Analyze physician suggestions and development improvement plans.

WOW Team

Focus: To develop the tools for staff to reward and recognize each other for living the values.

Task:

1. Develop and monitor the WOW card (staff recognizing staff) program.

MONETARY REWARDS FOR DESIRED PERFORMANCE

A number of institutions tie gain-sharing, bonuses, or outright gifting to patient satisfaction scores. Typically, satisfaction scores are in the "and if" category (e.g., "If profit exceeds one million and if patient satisfaction scores place us at least in the 75th percentile *vis a vis* our peers, then staff will receive . . ."). However, the number of hospitals and medical practices making patient satisfaction a *leading* criterion for monetary rewards is increasing.

Some institutions create a point system, with incremental points awarded for exceeding goals. Thus, in a hospital with a high managed care census, the staff bonus pool might be awarded one point if average length of stay drops to a particular number, two points if that number is even lower, and three points if it is below yet another level. Nosocomial infection rate goals might also be divided into three-point levels and so on with other desired and measurable outcomes. Patient satisfaction goals, too, may be divided into three-point levels. If the minimal target goal for an indicator is not achieved, then no points are earned by the staff for that issue. Points are totaled and each is worth a particular dollar amount in bonuses or profit sharing. Indicators may be differentially weighted or not.

Monetary awards need not be ongoing (e.g., annual). They can be one-shot to reward staff for having made unprecedented improvement.

Resist the temptation to test the waters by implementing a satisfaction-based monetary award program strictly for senior or middle managers. This can result in significant resentment on the part of nurses and other line staff who do the day-to-day job of treating and serving patients. If you want to start a monetary reward program piecemeal, then begin with the people who actually interact with patients and who are directly responsible for their care and satisfaction. If they earn their awards, then their managers deserve theirs—but not before.

As indicated earlier, monetary rewards are not essential. You do not need to institute big-buck profit sharing to motivate your staff. Symbolic rewards work. A personal note from one of the top administrators carries a lot of weight. Whenever top management visits staff and compliments them, whenever a recognition gift is given, whenever top management publicly lauds a department, unit, group, or individual, this constitutes a significant reward.

It cannot be stressed enough that if monetary awards are based at least partially on patient satisfaction, then you must provide staff with the training and opportunity to have a positive effect on scores *before* you begin using the data for this purpose. Otherwise, only frustration will result. Setting goals and dangling money in front of them does not help staff actually improve service. Do not confuse incentives with knowledge and techniques for improvement! Furthermore, be especially careful to base your reward structure on methodologically sound principles. For example, if you are a medical practice basing physician compensation or even employment on satisfaction survey results, then you must have a sufficiently large number of returned surveys for each physician to avoid basing action on spurious data.

Putting Some Teeth into the Program

It is relatively easy to enculturate new employees; they should be hired for patient-focused characteristics they already possess. But what about existing employees, from whom a patient satisfaction program may require new (and possibly threatening) modes of thinking and behaving?

Given the proper introduction, education, preparation, training, and implementation timetable, the vast majority of your existing staff will participate willingly and effectively in your program. However, participation cannot be voluntary—any more than proper hand washing can be left to individual choice. Without teeth, the program will not be taken seriously. If you mean business, then those who do not buy in cannot stay.

What makes a culture work and sustain itself is that its members *want* to behave as they *have* to behave. But first, you must clearly mandate the "have tos"—the required behaviors. Once your program is running and once sufficient, realistic buy-in time has passed, get rid of those whose unchanged attitudes and behaviors undermine your purpose and commitment. Patients who come into contact with these employees do not deserve less sensitive care than patients who interact with others—the vast majority—of your staff. Tolerating the noncompliant staff members' continued presence visibly suggests that you are not serious.

CONCLUSIONS

You are the hospital. Otherwise, it's just a building. Every individual must be trained to know this. Every individual has an impact on patient satisfaction. If not directly, then indirectly as a supplier of service to someone who does have direct access to the patient. Every person must be made to feel responsible for patient satisfaction

It is natural for staff to feel that they are already sensitive to the patient's personal needs and opinions. After all, healthcare naturally selects for such sensitivity, doesn't it? Nonetheless, staff must be reeducated in the principles of patient satisfaction and in the specifics of your improvement program. Staff must be primed and involved in the planning so as to develop ownership in and commitment to the program. The more clearly and specifically your satisfaction program is organized and scripted, the more chance of success.

Also, the more staff actively involved in the program, the more chance of success. Multiple teams or committees, as opposed to a single satisfaction committee, are advantageous because they broaden the scope of committed employees. If nearly all departments, units, or specialties have their own internal improvement teams, plus at least one member on a hospitalwide team, then it makes it more difficult for other department or unit members to opt out of the proper behavioral protocols. Such a strategy puts role models everywhere.

Offering monetary rewards to staff is not really necessary for high patient satisfaction. Rewards are a nice gesture, if you have the profit to justify it, and everyone can use an extra buck—but it is not essential. As we suggested in the second chapter, patient and employee satisfaction go hand in hand. When staff know they are satisfying patients, they justify and reinforce their own career choice. Healthcare professionals know that when their customers are satisfied, the result is far more significant than when commodity or other service customers are pleased with the product.

Priority concern for patient satisfaction is not an option for healthcare providers. In an increasingly competitive, litigious, and customer service–oriented economy, satisfying patients is as necessary as infection control and MRI maintenance. When patients are satisfied, what the hospital does to achieve its mission and ensure its survival is reinforced. There is no more cost-effective form of care enhancement, claim prevention, marketing, or employee morale building. When patients are satisfied with your care, they win, you win, your staff win, physicians win, and your payers win.

Patient satisfaction is good medicine.

And good business.

About the Author

A COFOUNDER OF Press Ganey Associates, Irwin Press, Ph.D., was the first to nationally promote patient satisfaction as both a component and indicator of healthcare quality. Since 1983, he has worked with hospitals across the country to implement satisfaction measures and improvement strategies.

Dr. Press received his B.S. in chemistry from Northwestern University, and his Ph.D. in cultural anthropology from the University of Chicago. Now Professor Emeritus, he taught anthropology at the University of Notre Dame since joining the faculty in 1965. He has conducted field research in Mexico, Colombia, Spain, and the United States, publishing widely on the clash between alternative ("folk" or "popular") medical practices and clinical ("official") medicine. His investigations into why patients use alternative healers rather than (or in addition to) physicians and formal medicine led to his winning a Lilly Faculty Fellowship and appointment as visiting professor at the University of Miami School of Medicine in 1980. There, he spent the year rotating through all clinical services at Jackson Memorial Hospital in Miami, Florida, observing interactions between patients and staff and recording patients' experience with clinical care.

Since founding Press Ganey Associates with Rodney F. Ganey, Ph.D. in 1985, Dr. Press has devoted himself to the task of making patient satisfaction measurement both practical and useful for physicians, hospitals, and other providers. He has served on the Quality Improvement Taskforce of the Joint Commission on Accreditation of Healthcare Organizations, and he was a member of the Research and Quality Improvement Council of the National Quality Forum. In 2004, he was named recipient of the first National Healthcare Consumer Advocacy Award by the Society for Healthcare Consumer Advocacy. A popular keynote speaker and workshop leader, he is widely recognized for his insight into the personal factors that affect the patient's experience and evaluation of care.